SPINNING STRAW INTO GOLD

□

Your Emotional Recovery

from Breast Cancer

□

RONNIE KAYE

Produced by Lamppost Press, Inc.

A FIRESIDE BOOK

Published by Simon & Schuster Inc.

New York   London   Toronto   Sydney   Tokyo   Singapore

Fireside

Simon & Schuster Building
Rockefeller Center
1230 Avenue of the Americas
New York, New York 10020

Copyright © 1991 by Lamppost Press, Inc. and Ronnie Kaye

Designed by Chris Welch
Manufactured in the United States of America

10 9 8 7 6 5 4 3 2 1

Library of Congress Cataloging in Publication Data
Kaye, Ronnie.
    Spinning straw into gold: your emotional recovery from breast
cancer / Ronnie Kaye.
        p.   cm.
    "A Fireside book."
    1. Breast—Cancer—Psychological aspects.   2. Mastectomy—
Psychological aspects.   I. Title.
RC280.B8K39   1991
616.99'44906—dc20   90-10238
ISBN 0-671-70164-9   CIP

. . . and when the girl was brought to the King he took her into a room which was quite full of straw, gave her a spinning-wheel and a reel, and said: "Now set to work, and if by tomorrow morning early you have not spun this straw into gold during the night, you must die." Thereupon he himself locked up the room, and left her in it alone. So there sat the poor miller's daughter, and for the life of her could not tell what to do; she had no idea how straw could be spun into gold. . . .

from the story "Rumpelstiltskin"

ACKNOWLEDGMENTS

It was only with the support and assistance of several wonderful people that this book became a reality. I would like to express my sincerest thanks to:

—Sivia Loria, for giving me countless hours of her valuable time. Her careful attention to structure and syntax was the magic that helped to transform the manuscript into a finished product.

—Shelley Kaye, for her constant encouragement, her endless patience, and her accurate and sensitive feedback.

—Jerry Bartlett, who gave me the space I needed, listened sympathetically to my frustrations, and kept me well-supplied with a steady flow of hugs.

—My agent, Roseann Hirsch, and my editor, Barbara Gess, for believing in this undertaking right from the start, and for their expert guidance along the way.

—The six women who formed my "advisory committee"—Gigi de Toledo, Alice Folkart, Chris Gulino, Elinore Ross, Juli Wasserman, and Sharon Zelle. All former breast cancer patients, these women provided me with a forum for discussing ideas and issues. Their valuable input helped to keep me on track.

—Three gifted physicians in the field of oncology, Armand Guiliano, Marilou Terpenning, and Michael VanScoy-Mosher, who reviewed the medical portions of the text and who believe whole-heartedly in the importance of treating the person rather than just the disease.

—Harriet Friedman, who helped me get "unstuck" many times and taught me to understand and appreciate my own creative process.

—The hundreds of women who have shared their deepest feelings with me and have allowed me the privilege of participating in their emotional recovery from breast cancer.

CONTENTS

INTRODUCTION

i lay on the examining table grinning, as my trusted gynecologist and I played an old, familiar game. For so many years, we had gone through the same routine. I would call the office and tell him that I had found a lump in my breast. He would ask me to come in just to make sure that it was nothing. Without fail, he would examine me, smile, and say, "Ronnie, go home. I'm sure this is nothing, but if it hasn't gone away after your next period, give me a call." I never called. There was never any reason to. The lump always went away.

So here I was again, on March 4, 1981, treating this as another excuse to visit with a physician that I have always liked and admired. As usual, Phil said, "Don't tell me where you found this lump. Let me examine you first. If, during the course of a thorough exam I haven't found it, then you can show me where it is." I closed my eyes to be absolutely sure that I wasn't sending out any clues. He began a gentle examination of my left breast, I felt myself smile inside. "Not there, Phil," I thought. Satisfied that there was nothing alarming on that side, he began to palpate my right breast. Suddenly the atmosphere in the room changed. I opened my eyes and saw the color draining out of his face. "Ronnie," he said, "this has to come out right away. Do you have a surgeon?"

I remember feeling terribly cold. The nurse brought blankets, and they piled them on top of me, as I lay there shivering. It was quite a while before they could stand me up on my feet. I was overcome with shock and a sense of unreality. "This cannot be happening to me," I thought. But it could, and it was. Phil was deadly serious about getting me to a surgeon as soon as possible. I found out only later that his mother had died of cancer very recently. He wanted me to live.

I have no recall as to how arrangements were made. All I know is there was such urgency that it seemed perfectly reasonable to be on the operating table less than twenty-four hours later. I knew nothing about breast cancer, much less about any options for treatment. The surgeon, while trying to reassure me, asked me to sign consent for a lymph node dissection, just on the outside chance that the lump turned out to be malignant. On the one hand, I did not believe his attempt to minimize the seriousness of the matter. On the other, I was still convinced, somewhere inside myself, that this was just a more elaborate game and that a reprieve would be forthcoming.

I vaguely remember a gurney, a lot of white, a very cold operating room, and a friendly anesthesiologist who held my hand when I told him how scared I was. The next thing I knew, I was waking up in what seemed to be a crib. I hadn't realized that bed rails are attached to hospital beds to keep patients from rolling off the side. I looked up into my husband's face and said, "What's the news?" He was silent for a moment. Then he answered, "Not as good as we had hoped." I felt an enormous dread welling up from deep inside. "What exactly does that mean?" I asked. "Ronnie," he said, "you have cancer."

I didn't know it then, but that was the beginning of the most incredible journey of my life. At the time, I had very little emotional energy to devote to worrying about breast cancer. Oh, I was definitely scared, and there was a period of time when I felt completely isolated and alone, but there were other pressing matters that demanded my attention. To begin with, I was finishing a graduate program in psychology and was in the process of studying for my comprehensive exams. On a personal level, my marriage was falling apart. In fact, my husband and I did separate a month after my treatment ended. At the same time, I had my hands full trying to deal with my two children, who were not only going through the standard teenage crazies but were also having a difficult time coping with their parents' divorce. I was determined to maintain my reputation as superwoman and had no intention of letting something like breast cancer slow me down. Accustomed for years to denying my feelings, I appeared to make a very fast and uncomplicated recovery, supported by the doctor's assurance that this had been caught early and I had no reason to anticipate anything other than a complete cure. In addition, I underwent a fairly new procedure called a "lumpectomy," which removed the tumor but saved my breast. I had to look very closely to see any difference between the way I looked before and after surgery. There was no blatant physical reminder that I had had cancer, which helped me get out of a marriage that really needed to end. Had I been unable to choose this procedure, had I lost my breast, I seriously doubt that I would have had the courage to leave the relative safety of my marriage. The social world of the single woman would have seemed totally inaccessible, and I would have been terrified that no man would ever want me.

And so, with my body pretty much intact, life went on. I passed my comprehensives and, shortly thereafter, began an internship at a local mental health clinic. Then, quite unexpectedly, my children, then aged fifteen and seventeen, decided to move out and live with their father. I experienced a devastating sense of loss. Struggling to establish an identity for myself independent of my roles as wife and mother, I sold my house and moved to the beach. I was alone, at the age of forty, for the first time in my life.

Gradually, I grew to like being on my own, having to please only myself, eating what and when I chose, staying up with a good book until three o'clock in the morning if I were so inclined, and concentrating on my career as a psychotherapist. I had just begun to truly enjoy my freedom when the unthinkable happened. One morning, while taking a shower, I slid a soapy hand over my right breast and discovered another lump. For hours I argued with myself about whether to call my surgeon. I knew that ultimately I would need to have this new lump checked, but my track record for having lumps that were "nothing" was no longer perfect. It had been only three-and-a-half years since my lumpectomy, and I was literally frozen with fear. However, the will to survive is surprisingly strong. Since I was too terrified to call the doctor, I did the next best thing. I called my closest friend and told her. "You call Dr. G—— right now, and then call me back," she insisted. "If I don't hear from you in ten minutes, I'm calling him myself!" So, of course, I called.

Beginning with that phone call, things started moving very quickly—biopsy, blood tests, X rays, scans. The verdict? The lump was malignant. With the recurrence of the disease, I had no choice but to undergo the complete removal of my breast—a mastectomy. There I was, forty-one-years-old, single, living alone, my entire family three thousand miles away. This time, I had no distractions to take my mind off what was happening. This time, I paid attention. I felt the fear, the terrible anticipation of a surgery which might save my life but leave me disfigured in a way I didn't know if I could accept, the dread of the return of a disease that might kill me—a flood of feelings so complex that I was totally overwhelmed.

When the surgery was over, I watched myself go through a period of physical and emotional recovery. The physical healing was rapid. What pain there was diminished quickly, and I did my prescribed exercises religiously to regain the full range of motion in my arm. In fact, exactly five weeks after I left the hospital, I was back on the slopes, skiing up a storm!

My emotional recovery was a different story. The road was long—almost ten months—and very hard. People looked at my exterior and decided that I was fine. I had no way of communicating the chaos that filled me—the grief, the anger, the terror, and the devastating feeling of loneliness. I had no idea where to turn. I was afraid to express the full range of my feelings, believing that there was too much inside me for any of my friends or relatives to bear. To make matters worse, sometimes I didn't even know what I was feeling; or, if I knew, I didn't understand why I was feeling that way. I desperately needed a role model—someone who had been through this and had dealt with it successfully, someone to whom I could pour out my heart and from whom I could gain strength and solace. I didn't know anyone like that. I needed to cry . . . and cry . . . and cry. Somehow, I just couldn't find a way to do that. I was so full of unshed tears that, at one point, I thought I truly might die.

But, as I said before, I am a survivor. Knowing that I couldn't remain grief-stricken, depressed, and filled with pain forever, I began to fight for my own recovery. I searched outside myself for people who were steadfast enough to tolerate my feelings and kind enough to treat me gently. I searched within, looking to connect with my core self, to reestablish feelings of self-worth, to question and redefine femininity, sexuality, acceptability, and beauty, and to come to terms with my own mortality. In the process, I learned more about myself than I had in years of therapy. I changed and grew in unexpected and very gratifying ways. I became more assertive, more self-assured, more open about my feelings, better able to ask for and accept comfort. I am a very different person today than I was at the time of my mastectomy, and I like the changes that have taken place. In a strange way, breast cancer has been one of the most valuable experiences in my entire life! I'm sure that must sound just a bit odd to most people, but the more breast cancer patients I meet and work with, the more I hear my own feelings echoed. A few years down the road, women who had done their homework look back and acknowledge that breast cancer was a critically important and extremely useful event in their lives.

As I was completing this process of recovery and growth, I found myself in the grip of two "isms" that seemed to occur almost simultaneously—professionalism and, for lack of a better word, altruism. There was a part of me that felt profoundly grateful that I had made it through this crisis in such good shape, and I was strongly motivated to act as a guide for other women. I wanted to save others some of the confusion, pain, and alienation I had endured. From the depths of my own experience, I could see a simpler, more direct route to recovery, and I was eager to share it with other breast cancer patients. In addition, as a psychotherapist, my professional self had become vitally interested in the potential value of this crisis, and in the opportunity for growth that lay hidden within the danger. In school, I had been taught that an acceptable goal in the area of crisis intervention was to return the patient to his/her previous level of functioning. Suddenly, that seemed like a terrible waste of a crisis. Why set our sights so low? Why not aim for maximum growth instead!

Driven by both the desire to give to others and the conviction that a crisis could be utilized to provide an incredibly powerful learning experience, I approached my local branch of the American Cancer Society with an offer to run an eight-week support group for breast cancer patients. That was five years ago. Since then, my groups have become an integral part of the service program. To date, I have worked with over five hundred women. In these groups, each woman has an opportunity to share her thoughts and feelings, her doubts and her deepest fears. She has a chance to listen to other women pouring out their hearts and to feel comforted by the fact that she is not alone. In a loving and supportive environment, the participants establish close contact with someone who has been there and now feels successful, joyful, and whole. With a model of what is possible before her, each of the women begins to create her own unique solutions to the problems she has brought to the group. The results have been most gratifying. The groups have been a pleasure to lead, and have proved very successful.

I am delighted that my work is making a significant difference in terms of a sound and rapid emotional recovery, but, for all those women I had been able to help, there were still thousands of others who were going through breast cancer experiences without the benefit of any kind of support or guidance, grappling with fear, confusion, depression, and grief basically on their own. I want to reach them, too. That's why I've written this book. In it, I can clearly define the many issues that arise and also present story after story of ordinary women and their extraordinary efforts to turn the crisis of breast cancer into a true opportunity for personal growth.

Although groups tend to be as unique as the individuals who attend them, the issues that arise seem to remain the same. The problems that women bring into group tend to repeat themselves over and over again, as do the feelings they experience. Based on my five years of work, I have compiled two lists—one of issues, and the other of feelings—and it is on these that the rest of the book is based. The issues include:

Death	Recurrence
Body image	Femininity
Sexuality	Isolation
Differentness	Fatigue
Communication	Treatment concerns
. . . with family/friends	Side effects
. . . with doctors	Relationship problems
Self-worth	

In addition to these important issues, women must also deal with a range of very strong feelings that are part of the normal response to a breast cancer diagnosis and treatment. The most common feelings are:

Fear	Vulnerability	Anger
Grief	Guilt	Sadness
Depression	Betrayal	Loneliness
Envy	Self-hate	Shame
Powerlessness	Anxiety	Resentment

I am certainly not suggesting that every item is relevant for every woman. It is, however, strangely comforting to find yourself somewhere on these lists and know that you are not alone—and that you are not crazy!

The book is organized into five basic sections. The first four chapters discuss the facts and feelings a woman must deal with from the time of diagnosis until surgery. Chapters 5–8 examine the specific concerns relating to surgical recovery and nonsurgical therapies. The next three chapters (9–11) are devoted exclusively to body issues. In Chapters 12–14, the many strong emotions that arise during and after treatment are explored. Finally, the last two chapters of the book

(15 and 16) study the ways in which a woman recovering from breast cancer relates to her world. Although the organization of the book is by no means arbitrary, I want to emphasize that there is no "right" order to what we feel. It must be made clear that anyone can feel anything at any time. Furthermore, there is always a very good reason for anything we feel, even if the reason is temporarily hidden from view.

My hope is that you find the rest of this book encouraging, reassuring, informative, supportive, and, most of all, challenging. I wish you a good journey.

ABOUT
DEATH

*W*hy begin a book on surviving breast cancer with a chapter about death? For two very important reasons: first, death from cancer is the most immediate fear that brings women into a breast cancer support group, and second, I thought it made sense to deal with the simplest issue first. Simple! What, you may ask, could be any more difficult than death? My answer, of course, is *Life*. But, you protest, other problems that come up have solutions. How on earth does anyone ever solve death? That is even simpler. Either you die or you learn to live with the fact that you are mortal . . . that one day, sooner or later, you will die.

The issue itself is no more complicated than that. However, the feelings that human beings in our Western culture experience as they wrestle with the fact of their own mortality are enormously painful— terror, fear of abandonment, anger, an overwhelming sense of un- fairness, and the kind of grief that makes one's throat ache. To be alive and suffer the loss of a loved one means that you have lost one person, no matter what he or she represents in your life. To con- template your own death means imagining yourself losing every- thing all at once—your family, your friends, your home, your job, your hobbies, your contact with the physical world, not to mention your own physical self.

It may seem impossible that anyone could make peace with such a personally devastating concept. Oddly enough, the thing that most often gets in the way of living comfortably with the notion of our own death is the fact that we all try so desperately hard to deny it. I have heard people refuse to purchase life insurance policies, lest they "jinx" themselves. This represents a kind of magical thinking common to young children who believe that the sun comes out because they open their eyes. In this case, the "ostrich syndrome" dictates that if we don't call attention to our existence by doing something foolish like buying life insurance, we might just live forever.

Given this hard-core denial of mortality, a woman who is suddenly confronted with the reality of a breast cancer diagnosis is likely to feel not only terror but sadness and loneliness as well. In a way, becoming aware of one's mortality for the first time is like losing one's innocence. And it is understandable when a person truly grieves for the loss of this innocence. Helping someone through this very difficult passage is best accomplished by one who has already made peace with the idea of her own death. Perhaps you will begin to understand how some resolution to this "unsolvable" problem is achieved as I share some of the experiences I have had, both personally and professionally.

Diane was a lovely forty-five-year-old woman who participated in one of my eight-week groups for breast cancer patients about two years ago. Her case was complicated. At the time, there was some indication that her cancer had spread, and her prognosis was guarded. When the group ended, I knew that there was a piece of work she had not completed. She was aware of it as well and requested some private time with me. In her first session, she filled the room with words. In the second session, she continued to talk on and on. At the beginning of the third hour she was strangely silent, and I asked her if she was finally ready to do her work. Looking pale and anxious, she nodded her head. As she sat in her chair, I asked her to close her eyes and move into the scary place that had been haunting her. Her eyes closed and she began to weep, filled with terror at the prospect of what was to come. I took her hand and told her that I would not abandon her, no matter what. And so, she began her journey.

"It's very dark," she said. "Very black and cold, like cement. And now I'm beginning to fall . . . down, down through the black— as if there's no end to the darkness." As she spoke, the tears were streaming down her face, and her hand was desperately clutching mine. "I have stopped falling now, and I am in a cave. It's very dark, and I am alone."

"How old do you feel as you stand in the cave?" I asked.

"Four," she replied. "I feel very small."

"Allow that four-year-old to speak," I said. "Let her tell us what she wants."

"I want my mommy," she cried. "I want her to hold me and make the black go away. I want her to make it all better."

I then suggested that she imagine her adult self joining that little girl in the cave to comfort her.

"As I walk into the cave," she continued, "I hold out my arms to her and she runs to me. I pick her up, wrap my arms around her, and gently begin to rock her."

"What is it you need to tell her?" I asked. "What is it she needs to hear from you?"

She thought for a moment and said, "I will always be with you. I'll never leave you."

"There's something more," I said. "One more thing you need to tell that child."

She sat silent, puzzled, not knowing how to continue. And then it came to her. "I love you very much," she whispered. In that instant, she felt the strong arms of her father, whom she had loved very dearly, encircle her and the child and embrace them, and she experienced a deep sense of peacefulness and well-being.

So ended the session.

When she returned the following week, she looked transformed.

"It seems," I said, smiling, "that you have finished your work."

"Yes I have," she said. "And now I'm ready to live."

This example illustrates many things. First of all, those fears you try to escape tend to pursue you with a vengeance. If only we had enough faith in ourselves to stand still for them, we would find that they dissipate in very surprising ways. Diane was terrified of confronting her own mortality, conceptualizing death in terms of a cold, black, and very lonely space. When she actually willed herself into that space, she discovered her own ability to comfort the child inside herself. Secondly, it demonstrates the extraordinary value of guided imagery. I often use imagery techniques with my patients because it allows them access to their "inner landscape" in a very unique and meaningful way. I spoke to Diane recently, and she told me that she can still feel the comfort and the peace that she first experienced in my office that day. And third, people who are frightened of death tend to talk about it in very similar terms: a black hole, a dark cave, a bottomless black pit, a black tunnel. For each representation, there is always the idea that there is no way out. While it is true that our efforts to avoid death are ultimately destined to be unsuccessful, we each possess the internal resources to make peace with our own mortality.

Obviously, in my line of work, I get to confront death on a fairly regular basis. People often ask me how I am able to stand it. I was fortunate to be able to spend six months in a group with terminally ill people. You might think this would have been terribly depressing. Quite the contrary, these were people who had faced the fact that their lives could end very soon and were invested in getting the most out of whatever time was left to them. They worked like demons to repair relationships, communicate love and caring, reach out in new ways, and take risks which they would never have taken before. I saw courage, but more than that, I saw joy. I watched people who were soon to die celebrate life and rejoice in their personal triumphs.

Sometimes, gaining a feeling of mastery over the terror of death requires little more than a change of perspective. I received a phone call a few years ago from a woman who sounded deeply distressed. Barbara had been diagnosed with breast cancer a year and a half before, underwent surgery, completed a six-month course of chemotherapy, and seemed to be doing well physically. Her complaint was that she couldn't stop crying. She was convinced that her cancer would recur and that she would die. Her family, on the other hand, considered her cured. After all, it had been such a long time since her illness. They believed her outbursts to be unreasonable and unpredictable, and they were beginning to question her emotional stability. There was talk about having her heavily medicated with antidepressants or even having her admitted to a psychiatric hospital. I invited her to attend a group, but she flatly refused. She felt very self-conscious, was uneasy about sharing herself with others, and believed herself to be such a desperate case that only a series of private appointments would do. So we scheduled a meeting at my office.

On the designated morning, I opened my door to find a pleasant-looking woman in her early fifties, slightly overweight, and dressed in the height of Los Angeles fashion—a designer sweatsuit. She appeared to be quite tense and anxious. When I invited her into my office, she plunked herself down on my couch, leaned forward, and said angrily, "I've never been in therapy before, and I don't like the idea at all! Just how long will this take?" "Eight weeks," I answered promptly. She sat back, stunned. She had thought that, because of the severity of her emotional state, she would have to undergo years of deep analysis. With that fear laid to rest, we began our exploration.

I asked her to tell me about these sudden, unexplainable bouts of crying. She recounted an incident that had occurred just recently. She had been working several days a week for her thirty-year-old son, whom she adored. On that particular day, he took her out for lunch to a very nice restaurant. Barbara was having a wonderful time, feeling loved and appreciating her warm connection with her son. In the middle of dessert, she suddenly began to cry so hard that she had to excuse herself from the table and run to the ladies' room, where it took her quite a while to compose herself. Of course, she was mortified. Both she and her family were convinced that these crying jags should have ended long before. After all, she had survived treatment. She was alive!

To me, this incident made perfect sense. Barbara was deeply attached to her husband and two children, and much of her life had been devoted to them. Every time she had a loving encounter with one of them, she was reminded that cancer had made her vulnerable, and she stood a chance of losing her connection with her loved ones.

The anticipated loss would cause a surge of grief accompanied by a flood of tears. Once she understood this, Barbara stopped worrying about being crazy and started asking how she could move past this point. One of the things we covered in that first session was the vulnerability of all human beings. Barbara had been blaming it on cancer, but, in truth, she could have stepped off the curb on her way home from my office and been run over by a bus. Vulnerability is simply part of the human condition. The other thing we discussed was the fact that each time we love, each time we commit to a relationship, we take a risk. The risk is that we could lose someone who has become important to us. Each of us can make the choice of loving and risking, or maintaining a "safe" distance and trying to insulate ourselves from the pain of loss. Barbara understood and chose, right then, to love.

We spent a very productive hour together. At the end of the session, as I was escorting her to the door, I said, "There's something I want to tell you before you go." She looked at me expectantly, waiting, I am sure, for the magic formula that would cure her instantly. "Barbara," I said gently, "I promise you that you will die." I watched as the shock registered on her face, then her eyes met mine and she nodded. "See you next week," she murmured.

A week later, she returned to my office with a smile on her face, a new hairdo, and, of course, a new sweatsuit. The first thing she told me was that she had begun a diet and a new exercise program. I commented that she seemed to be feeling quite a bit better this week, and asked if she knew why. "Well," she answered, "I think last week you reminded me of something I had temporarily forgotten. We all die sometime. I don't want to waste the rest of my life worrying about something that's inevitable."

Our next few sessions were spent reinforcing this new insight. We were also able to clear up some myths and misinformation about cancer, as well as some old patterns of communication that weren't working well anymore. Basically, however, the major part of the work had been done in the first two sessions. During her sixth session, I asked Barbara if she was ready to stop therapy. She acknowledged that she had gotten what she came for but wanted to come back for the last two sessions because she enjoyed our time together. Actually, she probably needed that extra support. Confronting mortality is frightening, and it can be reassuring to talk with someone who is truly comfortable with the issue.

Because no two people are exactly alike, each will find comfort in a unique way. Several months ago, I was privileged to work for a short time with a wonderful woman named Sharon. She was a kind and loving soul who, after her own recovery from breast cancer, had volunteered a great deal of time to bring hope and comfort to other women who were just beginning to go through the same experience. She had been troubled by a recurring nightmare. She was unable to remember it, but at the end of each dream she could see a vividly colored grid that terrified her, for reasons she did not understand. As we explored, we discovered that this grid was an image that had appeared in the hospital immediately after her mastectomy. There is a possibility that it was the first thing she "saw" when she came out of anesthesia. That connection explained the terror. The question was why this was occurring now, some three years after her treatment. It turned out that Sharon was being haunted by a statistic. Her doctor had told her that, without chemotherapy, she stood an 80 percent chance of recurrence within five years. If she agreed to undergo chemotherapy, it would reduce the chance of recurrence to 50 percent. Sharon had opted to undergo chemotherapy, but every day the five-year mark was getting closer, and she was growing more and more apprehensive. The statistics the doctor had offered with the intention of reassuring her were looming ominously. In short, she was afraid of death.

After we had done all the detective work, it was obvious that Sharon needed to directly confront her own fear. Using some hypnotic techniques, I asked her to see herself standing in front of the grid, and to imagine that a space gradually opened up so that she could walk through. Immediately, she saw herself running and had a sense of herself as a young and terrified child. She knew that she was being pursued by something awful, and that, if it caught her, she would cease to exist. As she continued to flee, I suggested that she had the power to put up a thick, impenetrable acrylic shield, colorless and perfectly clear of all distortions, that would separate her from whatever was chasing her. Once she had her shield in place, she would be able to study the unnamed terror.

Sharon quickly put up her shield and then turned around to face her pursuer. She saw what appeared to be a huge, black, hairy monster, who sat down quietly on the other side of the shield. From the moment she stopped running, Sharon could feel the terror lessening, even while she stood looking directly at the monster. After a few moments, I asked her to turn away from the monster and look behind her, where someone very safe and trustworthy was coming into her space—someone who knew exactly the right way to comfort her. She described a very large person whose face she couldn't quite see, who reached out and took her in his arms and simply held her. She reported feeling completely secure, and had no more worries about the monster that was still sitting behind the shield. The person then took her by the hand and led her out into the sunlight. The two of them walked off together, down a path where she saw the most beautiful flowers, all in vivid color.

The very second she came out of her trance, Sharon said, "I know who that person was. It was Jesus. When my connection with him is right, I feel completely secure. That doesn't mean I will never get sick, and it doesn't mean that I will never die. It just means that, no matter what happens, everything will be all right." Religion and spirituality had been an integral part of Sharon's upbringing. Over the previous few years, she had neglected that part of her life. Sometimes people forget that religious beliefs are not only valuable when things are going well, they are a source of great strength and comfort when life is difficult and challenging. That inner strength was still there, just waiting for Sharon to reach inside herself.

Religion as a source of strength may be right for some people and completely useless for others. The point of this chapter is that we all have the resources to make peace with mortality. Doing it is vitally important. How we do it is fascinating. There is no requirement that you use the same method or arrive at a resolution by walking exactly the same path that someone else has. However, the benefits of getting the job done are many. When you know that your time on earth is limited, each day becomes precious. You tend to do more of what you like, less of what you don't. It becomes a little easier to say no. It becomes more important to tell the special people in your life that you love them. Being judgmental or critical becomes a waste of time. Your perspective tends to change. Things that once seemed crucial become trivial, and the things that really matter become crystal clear. Coming to terms with death makes life much richer and more meaningful.

In the introduction, I pointed out that there is no prescribed order for feelings. They happen when they happen—and that is when they must be dealt with. Surprisingly, I didn't really come to terms with my own mortality until two years after my second surgery. Somehow, even though there were scary moments, or even scary weeks, I would always return to an optimistic view that this time I was truly cured. It is an interesting form of denial, and it worked . . . for a while.

One day, I received a call from a woman who had been in one of my groups a year before. Angela was a bright, dynamic, and attractive young woman who had added warmth, humor, and sensitivity to the group. She had very bad news. Her cancer had recurred and she was seriously ill. She wanted to see me, believing that I could offer her strength, comfort, and support. We set an appointment for two days later. When I hung up the phone, I could not stop trembling. For all my work, my encouragement, my insistence that women reinvest in life after breast cancer, a group member could still become terminally ill. My magic was gone—the magic that had been my own protective shield. I discovered that I was terrified of my own death.

Knowing that I must resolve my fear before I could be of any help to Angela, I turned to imagery. I sat back in a comfortable chair, focused on deep breathing, closed my eyes, allowed my body to relax completely, and waited for whatever internal picture might appear. Very soon the first scene began to unfold. I saw myself as a five-year-old clinging desperately to my mother and father. Before me there was a doorway filled with blackness. Through that doorway lay some unknown terror that, if I got sucked into it, I would have to face totally alone. I could feel myself being drawn by an almost magnetic force toward that darkness. Screaming and pleading with my parents to hold on to me, I tried to fight against that force, knowing always that, bit by bit, I would lose the battle and be lost in the void.

When the scene ended, I felt flooded with feelings of terror, helplessness, and great sadness. The day went by slowly, and that night I had a series of very disturbing dreams. Apparently, my unconscious mind was hard at work grappling with the issue at hand. The next afternoon, I once again sat back, closed my eyes, and waited. This time, a very different picture presented itself. There I was, a confident and self-assured woman, standing before a doorway filled with light. Feeling a wonderful sense of anticipation and excitement, I heard myself think, "Ah, that's the next place I get to explore." When I opened my eyes, all fear had vanished, and a sense of peace and security seemed to permeate my being. The fear has never returned.

I do not want to leave you with the impression that overcoming a fear of death or mortality can be accomplished in two days or that the issue can be resolved during the course of one dramatic experience in imagery. Most of the time, there is a great deal of preparation. One of the things I do with women who find themselves suffering from an unrelenting fear of death is to talk extensively about the subject. While talking does not solve the problem directly, it is very reassuring to know that something previously considered taboo can be discussed openly, especially when the person you are discussing it with is obviously not afraid. I would encourage you to find people who are comfortable with mortality and are willing to listen to your fears. Ask them to share their feelings and beliefs with you. It is amazing how effective openness can be in reducing the level of fear. Spend some time reading and rereading the stories in this chapter and in Chapter 14 (Living with the Fear). Although each person's story is different, the fact that every one of these women was able to resolve her fear of death can be reassuring. If they can do it, so can you.

While it is true that confronting mortality can be terrifying, it is also a challenge. It presents us with an invitation to address a multitude of important questions. What is death? Does death mean the end of consciousness? Is there such a thing as a soul? What about the idea of an afterlife? Is there another level of consciousness? A universal intelligence? God? I encourage the women I work with to explore these issues in depth. No matter if the exploration leads into unfamiliar territory. As you wrestle with these difficult concepts, you will eventually formulate your own belief system, one that will comfort and sustain you.

If you are willing to accept this challenge, there are many resources available to you as you search for your own answers. First, there are people, including members of the clergy as well as spiritual leaders and guides who are not associated with formal religions. Also, a multitude of books have been written on the subject. Appendix A has a list of suggested readings relating to this topic. The books I have recommended are not religious texts. Instead, they simply approach the questions of death and spirituality from many different directions. Not every book will appeal to every reader, but it is enlightening and reassuring to know that the issues can be approached and resolved in so many different ways.

When I deal with people who are afraid of death, I often find that they are unaware of significant contradictions in their beliefs. I recall a time when I was asked to come to the hospital to help a seriously ill woman deal with an almost paralyzing fear of death. When I asked her what she thought death was, she responded immediately, "Death is the end of all consciousness. After death, there is nothing . . . no sensation, no awareness, no thought . . . nothing. You simply cease to be." As we pursued the matter, I kept pressing her to tell me what was frightening her so. Finally, she sobbed, "It's scary to be all alone in the cold ground, with no one to hold me or comfort me." That certainly did not sound like the end of consciousness to me! I pointed out this contradiction, and in a relatively short time we were able to sort things out. I have met other people who insist that they have complete faith in repentance, absolution, forgiveness, and grace and yet cling to the belief that some "sin" they committed earlier in life is unpardonable. Again, this is a troublesome contradiction, and when it is cleared up the fear of mortality lightens considerably.

Most children have a tremendous fear of punishment and abandonment. These fears are so primary and so potent that they are often with us, lurking just out of consciousness, as we live our adult lives. Often, as we contemplate death, these early fears get mixed up with our current thinking and greatly complicate matters. In the last paragraph, the woman in the hospital was imagining death as a child would experience abandonment. People who are terrified of the consequences of some dreadful deed in their past are unaware that they are also grappling with a child's terror of punishment. Because it is so difficult for us to imagine no longer existing as the human beings we are, our considerations of death and mortality are often fraught with contradictions and projections of our childhood fears. Sorting this out can be done alone once we know what to look for. However, support and guidance can be extremely helpful at this time. If you find that you are having trouble dealing with these matters yourself, it makes good sense to have a few sessions with a therapist or counselor who has experience in this area.

Many times, people confuse other emotions with fear of death. Feelings of anguish, sadness, anger, or resentment about not being able to continue participating in life, or fear that your loved ones might not be able to survive without you are quite different from being afraid of death itself. These other feelings are also very normal and can be resolved as well, but it is difficult to come to terms with them unless you know what they are. I do want to stress that there is a big difference between resolving feelings and solving problems. Mortality cannot be solved. It is quite possible, however, to reach a comfortable level of acceptance of some of these unavoidable facts of life. Once again, if the sorting-out process seems too complex or confusing, or if the issues seem too profound or unmanageable, professional counseling can prove very valuable.

As I have illustrated in this chapter, I find imagery to be a wonderful way to deal with emotions on a very deep level. You will find many other examples of imagery throughout the book. If you have had previous experience with imagery, you can probably explore fears and concerns about death successfully on your own. However, if you are unfamiliar with the process, I would advise you to proceed with caution. I do not recommend that your first solo attempt at imagery be in this area. Because the subject of death is so frightening to so many people, there is always the possibility that you may suddenly confront a terrifying image and not know how to deal with it. For that reason, I strongly suggest that you pursue this with a guide who is not only experienced, but also well-versed in working with these particular issues.*

For those of you who are at the very beginning of a breast cancer experience, I would like to recommend that you put your concerns about death and mortality aside for now. There is so much to deal with at the time of diagnosis and in the beginning phases of treatment, that you need to focus all your attention on the day-to-day challenges that arise. Making peace with the idea of your own mortality is a process that takes time and effort. If reading this chapter has given you reason to believe that people can, in fact, arrive at some resolution, let that reassure you for now. Give yourself permission to address these issues at a time in the future when you have the opportunity to focus your full attention on them.

* Referrals for experienced guides and/or hypnotherapists in your area may be obtained from: The Academy for Guided Imagery, P.O. Box 2070, Mill Valley, CA 94942, 415-389-9324 (request their directory of imagery practitioners); American Society of Clinical Hypnosis, 2200 East Devon Avenue, Suite 291, Des Plaines, IL 60018, 708-297-3317. To request a referral list, send a self-addressed, stamped envelope.

FROM DIAGNOSIS TO TREATMENT

*i*t is frightening to be told that you have breast cancer, no matter who you are or how strong you imagine yourself to be. You suddenly feel alone, vulnerable, and very much out of control. A profound sense of shock—almost a type of paralysis—sets in. How long this feeling lasts is an individual matter. Some women snap out of it quickly and become actively involved in the pursuit of information and treatment options. Others remain confused and disorganized for varying lengths of time. Whatever your reaction, it is important to give yourself the right to feel whatever you are feeling, without any criticism or blame.

The time between diagnosis and treatment has been described by many of my patients as the most stressful period of all. In those first days or weeks after diagnosis, a woman is flooded with all sorts of information and opinions, not to mention wave after wave of terrifying thoughts and feelings. She must somehow pull herself together in order to fight most effectively for her own health and well-being. The emotional turmoil makes it very difficult to process facts and make intelligent decisions. It is important to understand that whatever you have felt or are feeling now, you are not unique. Thousands of women have felt the same way. As you read on, you will become familiar with some of the most common reactions other women have had. Facing these feelings, understanding them, and developing some perspective on them will make you feel less alone and help you navigate through the difficult and stressful time between diagnosis and treatment.

These are some of the statements women have made immediately following diagnosis:

1. "Cancer is a killer. No matter what anyone does, I know I will die a horrible death as a result of this."
2. "There has been a mistake. The doctors must be wrong." Or the alternative,
"This is a bad dream. I will wake up to find it's not real."
3. "Why has this happened to me? It's not fair!"
4. "The treatment will disfigure me, and no one will ever love me or want to be close to me again."
5. "The treatment is too difficult to endure."
6. "How can I make any decisions about treatment when I don't know the first thing about breast cancer?"
7. "I feel so alone."

The list goes on and on, but these are the feelings most often voiced. Because these issues come up on such a regular basis, it is worthwhile considering them one at a time.

I. CANCER MEANS DEATH

It is important to understand that **cancer is a diagnosis, not a death sentence!** Of course it is true that people die of cancer. If they did not, we would not be so afraid of it. But what so many women ignore is that people also *live* after being treated for cancer. Breast cancer, when discovered and treated in the earliest stage, has better than a 95 percent cure rate.

Many times, people hear a story about someone else, and immediately assume that the story is their own as well. The assumption may be false, but it is certainly human. For example, when I was a young mother, I learned that a neighbor's child had drowned in a swimming pool. All the other mothers in the area, myself included, were terrified for a few weeks. We felt very vulnerable, and jumped to the conclusion, at least temporarily, that one of our children would be next. It took a while for us to accept the reality that this very tragic story was not ours, and that just because it had happened to someone else did not automatically mean that it would happen to us. I use the term "boundaries" to refer to the fact that we are separate from other human beings, and have our own lives, our own stories, our own challenges, and our own outcomes. When we cross those boundaries, we tend to borrow other people's material, usually the sad and the frightening, and treat it as if it were our own. Most people know some sort of story about a person who has died of cancer. Remember, that is *a* story, not *your* story.

Unfortunately, many of us do not know anyone who has survived cancer. I must emphasize how valuable it is for the newly diagnosed breast cancer patient to meet and talk with women who have undergone treatment and now are happy and successful in their lives. These women are role models who can share their knowledge and experience with you about issues that, at the moment, seem insurmountable. It is highly appropriate to ask your doctor to put you in touch with some recovered patients who can guide you through the early stages of treatment. If that is not feasible, Appendix B lists several organizations that will give you access to recovered breast cancer patients who will be happy to talk with you before and after surgery. For example, the American Cancer Society has a volunteer group called Reach to Recovery. The members are former breast cancer patients who have been trained to make hospital and/or home visits to women who have just undergone surgery.* These same volunteers are also available to talk with patients even before surgery is per-

---

* The doctor or someone designated by him must contact the American Cancer Society to arrange a hospital visit by a Reach to Recovery volunteer. Patients may call on their own to request a home visit.

formed. A preoperative visit or phone call can be very reassuring. It is nice to know that, right from the start, you can have a connection with someone who has fully recovered, both physically and emotionally.

In May of 1988, I was privileged to speak at a European Reach to Recovery Conference. I have never forgotten the impact of walking into an auditorium where virtually all of the three hundred participants had had breast cancer. There were women from all over Europe, Australia, the West Indies, the Middle East, and the Americas. They were all vibrant, full of energy, and attractive and self-confident. There was a feeling of tremendous joy in that room. Never once did I detect a trace of apology or self-consciousness from those who had undergone treatment. They have a sense of great pride in who they are, what they have accomplished, and what they have to offer others. I often wish that I had videotaped that meeting. It would be absolutely clear to any woman viewing this scene that indeed there is life after breast cancer.

2. IT CAN'T BE TRUE

It is rare that a cancer diagnosis is a mistake, although it has been known to happen. However, the feeling that "it can't be true" is a very common reaction. Along with shock, denial may set in, at least for a while. While denial is not something we do consciously, it is actually one of the ways we attempt to protect ourselves from any kind of devastation. The unconscious mind says, "There is no way to absorb this dreadful news and still go on living. You need an adjustment period during which to believe that it cannot be true." Fortunately, in situations where there is a cancer diagnosis, this adjustment period tends to be extremely short. If a woman is to go through the necessary medical tests, work effectively with her doctors, make some very important decisions, and participate fully in all aspects of her treatment, she must first believe that her survival is indeed being threatened. The only time it seems reasonable to be concerned about denial is when it lasts long enough to put a woman's life in jeopardy. At that point, family, friends, or a physician must step in, and some counseling may be advisable.

It should be noted that denial is not limited to the breast cancer patient herself. When a loved one faces a breast cancer diagnosis, those who care about her experience their own distress. Sometimes they may insist that a mistake has been made. While their denial is understandable, their doubts must not interfere with proper care for the patient. Since close relationships can get fairly complicated, especially in times of stress, a consultation with a doctor, social worker, nurse, minister, or counselor might be extremely helpful.

Doubts about or a lack of confidence in one's doctor are very different from denial. It is important for you to feel that you are in good hands. If you are unsure, my suggestion is to get a second opinion. Many competent physicians encourage their patients to seek a consultation with another doctor and will help arrange one if asked.

3. WHY ME?

People, in general, try to understand the meaning of events in their lives, and get angry when things seem unfair or unjust. One of the questions I hear most often from the newly diagnosed breast cancer patient is, "Why me?" So many strong feelings are contained in such a simple question. Often women find themselves burning with anger at the unfairness of this crisis. Not all women are clear about where the rage comes from, which creates additional problems. We are all compelled to vent our anger somehow, and, when we do not understand the source of the anger, we tend to direct it toward innocent bystanders like spouses, doctors, nurses, children, friends, pets, or, even worse, ourselves. When everyone around you has become either a villain or an idiot, it is time to sit still and ask yourself what your anger is really about. When women have allowed themselves the time to observe and study their anger, they often find that there are other feelings underneath, like fear and sadness, which need to be dealt with. As these other feelings are confronted and explored, the anger tends to dissipate. Anger is a perfectly normal feeling, especially during the time between diagnosis and treatment. Abusing others or yourself because of that anger is simply not in your best interest.

Some women have a driving need to find some reason for their cancer. In an attempt to make sense out of this random and unjust event, they may come to illogical or erroneous conclusions. One very destructive approach is to assume that something you have done in your life was so bad that you deserve breast cancer—that, in short, life really is fair after all. Even if you have some incident in your past that you think is dreadful and inexcusable, read on. You will find stories of women in my groups who have been able to reveal such incidents. After being treated with the kindness and compassion they really deserved, they were able to shed lifelong burdens of guilt and shame. We all have our shortcomings. I do not know anyone who can boast of a past that has been filled with only good and generous deeds, charitable attitudes, and love for all beings. Few of us, however, are truly rotten to the core—and if you think you are one of the few, chances are you aren't!

Another unproductive way to attempt to understand the crisis is to tell yourself that you have never expressed anger properly, have kept your feelings inside, have stayed too long in a bad relationship, and so on. In short, you did not handle stress well. Then, not only must you contend with the cancer diagnosis itself, but also with the overpowering and self-imposed guilt of having caused your own disease. Many people are convinced that stress causes cancer. The truth is that no one knows exactly how stress relates to cancer. To date, the most that can be said is that chronic stress seems to have some impact on the immune system. That is not the same as saying that stress causes cancer. However, if you can identify sources of stress that you suspect are detrimental to your physical or emotional well-being, this can be a time to take stock, to reevaluate where you are in your life, and to make some changes. If you do this, the quality of your life is bound to improve. Whether or not stress is related to cancer, you will be happier, more fulfilled, and more powerful if you can lead a less stressful life. The message is quite clear. **Breast cancer is a challenge and an opportunity—not a punishment!**

4. DISFIGUREMENT AND FEAR OF REJECTION

One of the things a woman fears most as a result of a breast cancer diagnosis is that people will find her unacceptable—not just because she may lose her breast(s), but because she has a disease that others find terrifying. There is an appalling lack of information with regard to cancer in our society. Some people still believe that cancer is contagious. Several times, women have told me that they felt like lepers, and have been ashamed to let anyone know about their health status. A few of my patients have reported that, quite suddenly, friends had stopped hugging them! It is critical that your attitude toward yourself be kind, supportive, and very loving, for often the reactions you get from others are really reflections of your feelings about yourself.

Even if your self-image is quite positive, it is still possible that some of the people you know may turn away from you, at least temporarily. Even though it seems terribly rejecting, this has nothing at all to do with you. These are people who, for one reason or another, are so fearful and so threatened by what is happening to you that they find it impossible to face you and their own fears at the same time. To escape their fears, they may need to avoid you. Not only are they frightened, but they may also have difficulty finding the "right" thing to say. They feel responsible for solving this situation for you and find their own helplessness unbearable.

As you read through the chapter on communication, you will find many ways of dealing with these situations. You don't have to lose those who are dear to you just because of their initial reactions. On the other hand, it may be time to take a look at the people in your life. Ask yourself whether they love being taken care of by you but cannot or will not reciprocate. Are they too needy, too weak, or too self-centered to be supportive of you? If so, you may need to reevaluate the basis on which you form relationships. Many breast cancer patients have lived their lives believing that they must be superwomen and pillars of strength for everyone around them. The idea of receiving help or support from others may seem quite alien and disturbing. This may be an opportunity to revise your image in a very healthy way. Cancer pushes all of us to acknowledge that even we can be needy some of the time, and we too deserve to get our needs met.

When breast cancer is first diagnosed, it is often unclear whether or not a woman will have to lose her breast(s). If she is told that removal of a breast (mastectomy) gives her the best chance for survival, she is bound to feel trapped and fearful. Clearly, the decision should be made in favor of a long, cancer-free life. On the other hand, she may find herself wondering whether she will be able to live with herself after surgery, and whether anyone else will find her acceptable. Nothing is more terrifying than the unknown, and trying to anticipate how things will be after surgery is truly to imagine uncharted territory. Once again, role models are of utmost value. There are many women who have undergone mastectomies, are much loved by others, and feel wonderful about themselves. Meeting them and learning about how they resolved some of these difficult issues, can be especially meaningful during the time between diagnosis and treatment (see chapters on Body Image and Sexuality).

Finally, a word of caution. Beware of well-meaning people who make you feel guilty about your mastectomy concerns. In an effort to ease your pain, you may be told, "What difference does it make if you must lose a breast? Isn't your life more important?" Of course life is most important, but the loss of a part of yourself is important, too. You owe it to yourself never to allow anyone to trivialize your feelings. If you feel frightened, angry, sad, depressed, and are already grieving for this anticipated loss, you are experiencing what most women do at this time. Give yourself permission to have these feelings, because they are appropriate.

5. THE CURE IS WORSE THAN THE DISEASE

Some women find the thought of death easier to endure than the dreadful things they may have heard about breast cancer treatment. They imagine the very worst, and then question whether they could ever find the strength to undergo it. They fear surgery and its impact on their lives, anticipate terrible side effects from chemotherapy or radiation, and then envision themselves living forever after with the threat of recurring disease. It is important to understand that without treatment you will almost certainly be choosing death. In addition, if treatment were truly unendurable, it would never be offered to anyone. For most of us, life is very precious, and anything precious is worth fighting for. If you ask a fully recovered breast cancer patient whether treatment, no matter how uncomfortable or distressing, was worthwhile, you will undoubtedly be told that it was. While it may be difficult to have that perspective when you are newly diagnosed, it is very important to be in contact with women who are getting on with life and have their treatment behind them.

6. LACK OF INFORMATION

Part of the reason for the terrible confusion women experience during this period between diagnosis and treatment is that they know little or nothing about breast cancer. They are asked to make difficult decisions, cooperate in many tests that seem frightening and baffling, behave in a reasonable fashion, and appear intelligent and collected when they speak with their physicians, while, in reality, they simply do not know what is going on. In this situation, it should be clear that **knowledge is power**. The more you know, the better able you are to discuss your diagnosis and treatment with your doctor and to understand his answers! When you understand, you can become an active participant, *choosing* treatment because it is in your best interest. Having made the choice, you will feel much more in control, and much less like a victim. Knowledge is the most effective antidote to the bewilderment and disorganization that so many women feel at this time. You cannot expect yourself to magically acquire an advanced degree in medicine or biochemistry in the space of a week. However, there are many ways to become a well-informed layperson. There are several organizations that offer valuable resource material explaining the various aspects of breast cancer diagnosis and treatment (see Appendix C). A very basic explanation, designed primarily for those people who have no previous knowledge of the topic, can be found in Appendix D. If you wish to educate yourself on a more technical level, the medical librarian at your local university can help you do a search of the medical literature.

As you learn more, you may discover something rather dismaying. There are few hard-and-fast rules when it comes to breast cancer treatment at this time. Treatment may vary from woman to woman and from doctor to doctor. It is not unusual to receive differing opinions from even the most experienced and well-known physicians. This does not mean that some of the doctors must be wrong. It is simply a reflection of our current knowledge. Few treatment issues are black-and-white, and the gray areas are disturbingly large. Often women find this discouraging because they feel forced to make treatment decisions when they don't have the training or the background. It helps to know that there may be several different approaches, all of which are acceptable. Beyond that, it is very important to choose a doctor in whom you have confidence and with whom you can imagine working closely over the months to come. It is preferable to select a doctor who will answer questions graciously and explain tests and procedures along the way.

There are times when the shock and confusion are so profound that even the most competent of women find themselves unable to absorb any technical information. Some time ago, I received a phone call from a member of my ski club, who told me that a good friend of his had just been diagnosed with breast cancer. He felt that a call from me would be very reassuring to her. I had been acquainted with Charlene for many years and knew her to be a strong, capable, no-nonsense type of person. She held a high position as administrator and instructor at a professional school, and her ability to organize herself and everyone around her was impressive. As I dialed, I was certain that she would already have taken complete charge of the situation, and that my call would simply be a friendly gesture. Much to my amazement, she could barely talk, and kept muttering, "I can't think . . . I don't understand." Fortunately, she had a friend with her who was willing to take her to the doctor for a question-and-answer session. I asked the friend to get pencil and paper and proceeded to dictate a long list of questions to ask during the consultation. The questions were organized in such a way that, as one answer followed the next, a simple but complete picture of the situation would begin to emerge. Since Charlene might still be too disoriented to assimilate any of the details at that point, I suggested that they bring a tape recorder, so that she could review the session later, at her leisure. I called the next day to check up on her. She sounded steady, much more in control, and ready to mobilize herself. By breaking the information down into easily digested pieces, Charlene had been able to come out of her shock a little at a time, until she felt capable of taking charge. Tape recorders and written lists of questions can be helpful all through the process of treatment, but are especially valuable in the early days. (A sample list of questions will be found in Appendix E.)

7. FEELING ALONE

Although you can be surrounded by the most loving family and friends, chances are there will be times during diagnosis and treatment when you will feel profoundly alone. There is no contradiction here. No matter how much support you get from others, you are the one facing this disease, and you are the one fighting for your life. I was hit by waves of aloneness as I moved through my own treatment and recovery and have heard one patient after another echo this experience. Several months ago, a very poignant incident occurred that illustrates this feeling.

My mother phoned to tell me that something suspicious had been found on her mammogram. Although we live three thousand miles apart, we were in close touch from that moment on. Giving her the benefit of all my personal and professional experience, I explained medical terms, found doctors, and encouraged her as best I could. She did, in fact, have breast cancer, but it was discovered so early that treatment was fairly minimal. A few weeks later, I asked her whether having had access to me had made any difference to her. "Not really," she replied. I was astonished! Of course I had expected to hear a resounding YES, especially after all my talk about role models and group support. When I asked her to elaborate, she said, "Well, it was good to have you there, and I was glad that you could explain things and help me choose a competent doctor, but . . . *it was happening to me!*" How those few words touched my heart! I knew, from the depth of my own experience, exactly what she meant. Ultimately, she was alone with the diagnosis, she would be the one to undergo treatment, and she was the one whose life was being threatened. Nothing I had to contribute, no matter how valuable, could change those facts.

While there is nothing that can change the truth of how you feel, communicating it to others who understand helps to lift the heaviness of it. One of the benefits of being in a group is discovering that others are feeling similar pain. This establishes a common ground of shared experience and a sense of connectedness that will permit the cloud of loneliness and isolation to dissipate.

chapter three

. . . AND DO YOU HAVE A TEDDY BEAR?

*Y*ears ago, when I had just started out as a psychotherapist in private practice, I began to notice an interesting phenomenon. Again and again I observed that patients went through sessions where they actually appeared to be young children. Voices grew squeaky and high-pitched, postures changed, tears seemed closer to the surface, and people seemed much more connected with their feelings. At those times, my patients seemed to be sharing themselves with me in a deeper and more authentic way, and I always found myself profoundly moved. Then, one day, while working with a patient on an issue that was totally unrelated to cancer, I had an experience that aroused my fascination with what I came to call the "inner child."

Vince, a tall, ruggedly handsome young man in his early thirties, had been working with me for several months. On this particular day, he came to my office red-faced and yelling. His girlfriend had been having some contact with her ex-husband. When Vince insisted that she stop, his girlfriend accused him of trying to run her life. Vince had then asked his friends whether they would put up with her outrageous behavior, and they had unanimously agreed that they would not. He spent the first fifteen minutes of the session angrily attempting to justify his position, and trying to convince me that he had a very legitimate complaint.

I listened patiently, giving him the opportunity to vent some of his rage. When he had finally talked himself out, I said very gently, "Vince, imagine that you are four years old, having this same experience. As a four-year-old, what would you really be saying?"

I watched, enthralled, as he grew very quiet, his breathing slowed, his shoulders, which had been raised and very tight, drooped, and a suspicious glint of moisture appeared in his eyes. He said softly, "I'm so scared that there won't be enough love left for me." After a moment, he pulled himself together and exclaimed, "That's ridiculous! I can't imagine where that came from. I should never say anything like that. In fact, I should never feel anything like that!" It took me a while to calm him down again. I let him know that his simple, unadorned, undefended way of communicating had touched my heart in a way that his anger never could. I encouraged him to go back to his girlfriend and communicate to her directly from that four-year-old part of himself. He was a bit doubtful when he left, but, since his old methods had proved so unsuccessful, he was willing to try something new.

Vince returned to my office the following week looking happy and a bit puzzled. No sooner had he told his girlfriend exactly what we had discussed, than she had thrown her arms around him and assured him that he meant more to her than anyone in the world. She explained the reason for her contact with her ex-husband and began to explore ways to accomplish what was necessary without making Vince feel threatened. Vince told me that his bad feelings had disappeared just as soon as she had heard him, hugged him, and reassured him. He was amazed that one very simple sentence coming directly from his "inner child" had accomplished what a week's worth of anger had failed to achieve.

As the years went by, I often used the idea of the "inner child" in my work with patients. They found it enormously helpful, and so did I. It seemed to give us access to psychological and emotional material that had previously been beyond reach. At that time, however, I still felt that asking a patient, "How old do you feel right now?" was simply a technique that worked well and yielded positive results. I had no reason to think about whether that "inner child" was real or not until I had my own personal experience with it.

The night before my mastectomy, my mother, my daughter, and several friends had come to the hospital to spend some time with me. A bizarre party atmosphere pervaded the room. No one talked about the "event" that was scheduled for ten o'clock the next morning. The people around me were trying hard to keep things light. It was a strange interlude, where nothing real was brought up by anyone else, and I felt too self-conscious and vulnerable to do it myself. Suddenly, as if there had been some silent communication among the visitors, everyone stood up, said their goodbyes, and left. Nine o'clock, and I was alone. I felt almost suffocated with fear.

Woodenly, automatically, I began to go through the motions of getting myself ready for bed, when I noticed a little white teddy bear sitting on my pillow. He had been left there by one of my friends. On impulse, I took him in my arms and curled up on the bed. Ten minutes later, there was a knock on my door, and a doctor walked in. I sat up quickly, trying as best I could to disguise the fact that I had just been caught hugging a stuffed bear.

"Hi," he said. "My name is Dr. M——. I will be your anesthesiologist tomorrow. I stopped in to see whether you have any questions about the procedure."

Suddenly my eyes filled with tears, and without a moment's hesitation I asked in a very shaky voice, "Could I keep my bear with me?"

Dr. M—— studied me intently for a few seconds, then flashed me one of the kindest smiles I have ever seen and said, "Don't worry. I'll work something out."

His response made me feel better. He had heard my distress, and had responded to it in a humane way—no questions, no criticisms, no judgments.

The next morning, I kept my bear with me as I was wheeled down to the operating room. I spotted Dr. M—— immediately. He came over, took my hand, and flashed me another one of his wonderful smiles accompanied by a conspiratorial wink. He hadn't forgotten. Soon I was asleep, and the mastectomy was in progress. I awoke in the recovery room a few hours later feeling as though I had only been out for ten minutes. Looking down, I saw the teddy bear tucked securely under my left arm, with one of my hospital identification bracelets around its neck. That bear instantly became a very important personality in my life. I named him simply my "hospital bear," and I slept with him tucked under my chin for almost six months after my surgery. Now, years later, I loan him out to patients who need him. To this day, I am grateful to that wonderful doctor for recognizing my right to feel like a young and very frightened child and to be comforted accordingly.

Once I had recovered, I began to give a great deal of thought to the teddy-bear incident. I wondered whether the "inner child" might not be more than just a therapeutic tool. I was certainly not acting when I asked the doctor about my bear. I seemed to have actually become a very young child. I felt her feelings and spoke with her voice. There was nothing premeditated about it. That child was me, and I was that child. Intrigued, I started to explore the notion of the "inner child" and finally arrived at some conclusions about how we, as human beings, are organized psychologically and emotionally.

What exactly is the "inner child"? The best way to understand it is to observe people's behavior over a period of time. You will notice that, at any given time, a behavior will always fall into one of three distinct categories: Parent, Adult, or Child. Actually, these are more than just categories. Parent, Adult, and Child are three ways of being—each one clearly identifiable by certain gestures, expressions, and mannerisms. The Parent is made up of behaviors copied from parents or authority figures, and holds society's traditions and values. When there is a need to nurture or protect, to control or to criticize, it is the Parent that goes into action. When a person is operating from the Parent state, you might expect to hear things like this:

"You should always respect your elders."

"Did you hurt your knee? Here, let me kiss it and make it all better."

"Come in here this minute! You must *never* ride your bicycle in the street!"

The Adult functions basically as a computer. It processes facts and comes to logical conclusions. A person who is operating from the Adult is in a problem-solving mode and is temporarily out of touch with emotions. Filling out a tax return, cutting a dress pattern, or trying to anticipate how much food will be needed to feed a crowd of twenty are the types of behavior that fall into the domain of the Adult.

The Child is the part that gives people access to feelings such as joy, sadness, anger, and fear. It is the part that processes life's events on an emotional level. It is also the part that holds emotional memories from the past. If you want a direct experience of your own Child, take a ride on a roller coaster, eat an ice cream sundae, play with some modeling clay, or watch a scary movie. If you want to observe someone else in this Child state, go to a football game and watch an avid fan. You'll see lots of emotion—enthusiasm, disappointment, anger, joy—all of which will have an obviously childlike quality. The Child is the gateway to creativity, fun, sexuality, and freedom.

Ideally, people should be able to move freely from one state to another, selecting the mind-set and the behaviors that are most appropriate in any given situation. Unfortunately, in the process of growing up, we are taught that emotions get in our way—that they are not useful in the real world. In order to gain approval, we learn to cover up those emotions. To protect ourselves from criticism and rejection, we bury our feelings and try to appear rational. The Child, which continually sends us messages about our emotional needs and desires, is forced to go underground. This is the origin of the "inner child." The trouble is that the "inner child" will not give up. If we don't attend to the direct messages we are sent, the communications will start coming through in code—headaches, ulcers, neck and back spasms, depression, anxiety, and many other attention-getters that we call symptoms.

Think of a time when you were under tremendous stress or felt very threatened. Ask yourself how old you felt at that moment. Chances are you felt quite young. People are often surprised the first time they recognize the child within themselves. The "inner child" remembers danger, abandonment, loss, grief, fear, and rage because it has experienced those emotions in the past. When current situations bear even a remote resemblance to past events on an emotional level, the "inner child" is mobilized. Whenever the "inner child" is flooded with powerful emotions, there is a pressing need to have those feelings heard and acknowledged. Once the "inner child" perceives that the message is getting through, there is likely to be a request for action of some kind. Have you ever wished that someone would hug you when you were feeling upset? That was your "inner child" asking for comfort.

Wishing for a hug is one thing, but letting someone else know that you *need* a hug is quite a different matter. Somehow, many of us come to believe that being adult means we must be strong, independent, and self-sufficient at all times. We try to act as if we are too old to long for comfort and reassurance when things get rough. That may work well enough when life simply goes along as usual. However, during a crisis the "inner child" really clamors to be heard. The need for comfort becomes very strong and very immediate. We become vulnerable, and we have learned to find that embarrassing and immature.

We are often afraid to pay attention to the "inner child." The feelings contained within us seem so powerful, our longings and needs so immense, that we fear we would be totally overwhelmed if that Pandora's box were ever opened. Nothing could be further from the truth. When it comes to feelings, the simple fact is: **what you ignore will pursue you!** If you refuse to pay attention to what you feel, that feeling becomes the psychological equivalent of a hungry wolf. The faster you run, the harder it chases you. On the other hand, if you have the courage to stand still and face what you feel, the strength of that feeling will tend to diminish in a relatively short period of time. Standing still for your feelings has some other advantages too. You may learn something about a part of yourself that you have ignored for years, and once you are able to understand the feelings and needs of your "inner child," you can get those needs met. When your "inner child" is truly cared for, you will experience a wonderful sense of well-being and freedom.

Getting in touch with your "inner child" is a relatively simple matter. If you are struggling with feelings or reactions that you are finding difficult to understand, ask yourself the following: "How old do I feel right now?" If you can't respond to that directly, you might ask, "If I were to imagine myself as a child right now, how old would I be?" Some people find it difficult to relate to a specific age, but are able to imagine themselves as a young child. That approach is just as productive. Then, once you have identified or imagined that child, continue the process by asking, "As this young child, what do I really have to say about my situation?" At this point, it is your job to pay attention to the communications you receive. They may come through as feelings, images, words, thoughts, or some combination of these. Don't screen anything that comes up, and don't judge the material as good or bad. Simply treat whatever surfaces as valuable information about your feelings and needs at this time. Once your "inner child" is communicating with you in some fashion, the next question which must be asked is, "As this young child, what is my most immediate need?" The most common responses include the need to be hugged, held, cuddled, rocked, comforted, talked to, reassured, or protected. If the need you uncover is fairly general, it is important to pursue it so that you wind up with specific details. Two people who have a need for protection might want that need satisfied in entirely different ways. If, on the other hand, your need is already specific, like the need to be hugged, the only other question to be asked is "By whom?" When you decide to establish a connection with your "inner child," make sure that you are in a quiet, comfortable environment where there are no distractions and no demands being made on you. Although the process is a simple one, it requires some focused attention at first.

Another wonderful way to reach your "inner child" is through imagery. In the back of this book, you will find a Relaxation and Imagery Supplement that explains some very basic imagery techniques and provides a simple script to follow if you wish to have a dialogue with your "inner child." If you are interested in teaching yourself imagery on a more sophisticated level, I highly recommend a book by Martin L. Rossman, M.D., entitled *Healing Yourself.* Dr.

Rossman expertly leads the reader through the early phases of imagery and then introduces some of the more advanced concepts and techniques. In addition, he has produced a set of accompanying audio tapes* for people who would feel more comfortable having an experienced "guide" to help them at first.

Over the years, I have taught women in my breast cancer support groups how to connect with their "inner child." I have invited them to communicate with the group directly from that part of themselves, conveying their fears and hurts to people who can listen with compassion. It is always amazing to see what happens after these feelings are expressed and the much-needed comfort and reassurance are obtained. A case in point is Loretta, a soft-spoken, elegant, and very refined woman in her mid-sixties. When she first came to my group, she sat as still as a stone, never sharing anything except her name. I know that being in a group can sometimes make people feel threatened, so I never demand that they participate, but I do gently encourage them to do so whenever I can.

Three weeks went by, and, although Loretta showed up promptly for every meeting, she sat silent while other group members spoke. In the fourth session, I asked her whether she was getting what she needed for herself, even though she was not speaking up. Suddenly, a look of fear appeared on her face. She swallowed hard several times, unable to get any words out. Finally she whispered, "I would like to talk, but I am really terrified." Gently, I asked the familiar question, "Loretta, how old do you feel right at this moment?" Tears began to trickle slowly down her face. "Six years old," she replied, "and I have been beaten very badly for telling people how I feel." Everyone in the room was overcome with feelings of compassion and protectiveness. I looked at Loretta, and quietly said, "No one in here will ever beat you for expressing what you feel. My commitment to the group is to make this space absolutely safe for any and all emotions." Around the room, heads nodded vigorously.

* Rossman, Martin L., M.D. *Healing Yourself.* Pocket Books: New York, 1987. Both the book and the audio tapes are available from Insight Publishing, Box 2070, Mill Valley, CA 94942, 1-800-234-8562.

When Loretta looked around, saw the support and heard the reassurance, she knew that her "inner child" had been recognized and validated. Within a very few weeks, she became one of the group's most active members, able to bring up issues that were of concern to her and to receive the support she needed.

As my work with breast cancer patients continued, I came to understand that focus on the "inner child" was truly an integral part of recovery. I incorporated it into my practice, stocking my office with teddy bears and encouraging patients to connect with that part of themselves. One day, I had an opportunity to use this approach over the phone with a woman I had never met before. It was an unusual call right from the start.

"Hello," she said. "My name is Janet. I really don't know who you are or what you do. I got your name from a nurse at the hospital where I'm scheduled to have surgery for breast cancer in two days. She seemed to think you might be helpful."

She sounded so forlorn that my heart went out to her. "Well," I responded, "perhaps we can figure out what your most immediate need is, and we'll go from there."

There was a moment of silence and then she said tearfully, "Can you help me make out a list? I don't know what to take with me to the hospital."

Although I was much more accustomed to being asked about emotional and psychological issues, I understood that Janet was having a difficult time getting herself organized in any way. Quickly reviewing my own experiences in hospitals, I began to formulate a list designed to anticipate any needs that might come up during her hospital stay. The list included everything from her own bar of soap (hospital soap can smell pretty medicinal) to the type of clothes she would be comfortable coming home in. One by one, I ticked off those items that I thought would make her feel as though she were taking care of herself in every conceivable way.

When I had run out of suggestions, I paused for a moment and then, quite spontaneously, added, ". . . and do you have a teddy bear?"

"A teddy bear?" she repeated, sounding a bit shocked. "Why do I need a teddy bear?"

"Because," I replied with certainty, "it's a nice thing to hold on to when you're scared."

"But I don't have one," said Janet. "What do I do now?"

"When do you check into the hospital?" I asked.

"Tomorrow afternoon at four," she answered.

We went over the things she had to do the next morning, and figured out that she had some time early in the afternoon to buy herself a bear. I also told her that there would be a breast cancer group starting in three weeks, and invited her to attend. That was the end of our conversation.

Three weeks later, sitting around a large conference table at American Cancer Society headquarters, I asked the members of my new group to introduce themselves. We got halfway around the table when a familiar voice said, "My name is Janet, and I spoke to you over the phone a few weeks ago. I want to thank you. When everyone else was telling me strange and frightening things, you told me about teddy bears. I did go out and buy a bear. I did take him with me to the hospital. I did take him down to surgery with me. My doctor, who had been very stern and uncommunicative right from the beginning, looked over and said, 'I see you have a bear.' I asked him in a very quavery voice whether I could keep the bear with me until I was asleep. Gruffly, he answered, 'Well, I suppose so.' When I woke up in the recovery room, my bear was propped up next to me on my pillow. As my eyes slowly began to focus, I saw a nurse bustling around the room. Her efficient, no-nonsense manner reminded me of a drill sergeant in the army. As she walked toward my bed, I was sure I was in for a rough time. Much to my surprise, she leaned over and said, 'Oh, that's a very nice bear. I have several just like it in my collection. It's a very good brand, you know.' That bear has done his job well. He really protected me."

The following week, when the group reconvened, I asked whether anything that related to our previous session had come up during the week. A very chic and lovely Frenchwoman in her late fifties raised her hand and, in the most delightful accent, said shyly, "I went out this week and bought myself a bear!"

chapter four

□

SURGERY AND THE FEAR OF THE UNKNOWN

*a*s the time between diagnosis and treatment draws to a close, most women find themselves preparing for surgery. For some, the procedure will leave their bodies pretty much unchanged, while for others, removal of one or both breasts is necessary for the best chance of cancer-free survival. Regardless of the type of surgery performed, the lymph nodes under the arm are usually removed (see Appendix D). These procedures take place in the operating room under general anesthesia. The closer surgery gets, the more anxious and fearful one tends to become. These feelings are absolutely normal. After all, no matter how "minor" or "routine" the surgery may be to anyone else, it is always major if you are the patient.

There are several reasons for the fears and concerns which surround surgery. The best discussion I have heard on the topic took place in one of my breast cancer groups. One evening, several group members had gotten onto the subject of the "befores and afters" of surgery. It had been a time filled with fear, anger, helplessness, and vulnerability, and the women now needed to have their feelings about it heard and understood.

MICHELLE: I was petrified. From the moment of my diagnosis, all I could think about was that all my life cancer had been such a dirty word. I was afraid they would open me up, find me full of cancer, and give me up as hopeless.

JANET: My first concern was whether I would wake up at all! My doctor told me that there was a risk of dying because of the anesthesia, and then handed me a paper to sign indicating that I understood. I felt as though I were being asked to sign my own death warrant!

RONNIE: I think you may be referring to something we call "informed consent." There is a law that says patients must be fully informed of all risks before they agree to any procedures.

JANET: I know that now. But it was said so matter-of-factly. I could have used some compassion at the time. After all, the doctor and I both knew that I had to have the surgery. Without it, I would surely have died of cancer. I agree that I should have been informed, but I didn't have to be scared to death!

BLAIRE: The two things that scared me the most before surgery were how much pain I might have and how I would look afterward. Although I was terribly afraid, at least I could tell myself that anyone in my position would probably be feeling the same thing. What I wasn't prepared for was the series of shocks I experienced after surgery was over. First of all, the surgeon had never told me about the size or location of the scar, or the fact that I would have a drain hanging out of my side. I didn't expect to see a red line extending from the middle of my chest all the way across and under my arm. Then I found that I couldn't raise my arm at all. Naturally, I panicked and rang for a nurse. She explained that it is normal to have limited range of motion after this kind of surgery. She was the one who told me about the exercises I would need to do. On top of all that, I discovered that I was numb in my armpit and along the back of my upper arm. By then I was really frantic. I thought that meant that the cancer had spread. When I found out that this numbness is due to the nerves that are cut during surgery, that it's pretty typical, and that it might be permanent, I was outraged. This was another loss that I hadn't bargained for.

MICHELLE: Now that I think about it, the other thing I had

trouble with was the hospital itself. The only times in my life that I had ever been in surgery were to give birth to my three children. On those occasions I was so focused on myself and the happy reason I was there that I really didn't have time to think about anything else. This time, waiting for a surgery that was frightening to begin with, I realize how lost I felt in the hospital routine. Every moment there was something else that was unfamiliar and potentially threatening. I never knew what was going to be coming at me next. The unknown is really very frightening.

As I heard that last sentence, I thought back to a time about four months after my first surgery. My radiation treatments had ended, and I thought I had put the whole experience behind me. Then I got a phone call from a long-time friend, Audrey, whose mother had died of breast cancer many years before. Audrey had found a lump in her breast that the doctor thought was suspicious. She was scheduled to have a biopsy in two days. The surgeon had insisted that the biopsy be performed under general anesthesia, on the chance that the lump was malignant. That way, he would be free to perform a lymph node dissection at the same time. With the added burden of her family history, Audrey was understandably terrified. When I offered to go to the hospital with her, she accepted without a moment's hesitation.

By some strange coincidence, Audrey was going to be admitted to the same hospital I had been in, the procedure she was about to undergo was identical to mine, and her surgeon was the same one who had performed my biopsy just a few months before. From where she stood, everything was unknown. Audrey was looking to me as the expert, because, as she said, I knew the ropes. Because of my personal experience, I was familiar with the whole routine, and was certainly well qualified to run interference for her. I was determined to do whatever I could to alleviate her fear.

The morning of surgery, I met Audrey and her husband at the hospital. As we sat in her room, I began to explain the time schedule. I told her about the injection the nurse would administer to relax her. I described the trip to the operating room and the place where she would wait until one of the operating rooms was free. I recommended that she ask for extra blankets when she got to the recovery room after surgery, because they keep that room very cold. I introduced her to the anesthesiologist, a man I had known for many years, and helped to create a friendly connection between them. I let her know that some nausea after surgery is quite normal and that it passes fairly quickly. I also told her approximately how long she would have to wait for the preliminary pathology report that would tell her whether the tissue which had been removed was benign or malignant. I shared every bit of my own knowledge and experience with her, hoping that this would alleviate some of her fear. I remained until Audrey was wheeled down to surgery. Before I left, I asked her husband to call me when she got back to her room and the pathology report was available.

Late that afternoon, I was preparing dinner for my family when the phone rang. It was Audrey, calling to tell me that the procedure had gone well and that the lump was benign. She thanked me for my efforts, saying that she had felt much more secure just knowing what to expect at each turn. We spoke long enough for me to congratulate her on the good news, and then hung up so that she could get some rest. No sooner had I gotten off the phone than I burst into tears. It took me a while to understand this very unexpected reaction. First, I was able to connect with a part of myself that felt angry, envious, and resentful. I could hear a voice in my head shrieking, "It's not fair! Why me and not her?" How I wished that I, too, could have been one of the lucky ones—one of the women who gets to go home with a clean bill of health. It took a little longer for me to hear yet another voice. This one sounded much more like a forlorn child crying despairingly, "I needed protection, too. When I was feeling so alone and so frightened, why wasn't there someone to give me what I had given to Audrey?" I hadn't realized until that moment how terrified I had been of the unknown.

There are many things a woman can do to deal with the unknowns surrounding surgery. It can be very helpful and reassuring to speak with someone who has been through a similar procedure, especially if she has made significant progress in terms of her own emotional recovery. However, we tend to ignore some of the best resources available—namely, the health professionals with whom we come into contact during this period of time. If only we knew what questions to ask, we could get answers from our surgeons, from their support staffs, including nurses and technicians, and from the nurses on the surgical floors in the hospitals. If more practitioners knew how fearful women are before surgery, they could find ways to provide access to some specific information that might well allay many of those fears. With no feedback, doctors can assume that their patients are doing well. Unfortunately, many women are reluctant to express their concerns to their physicians. They worry about being judged as too troublesome, too demanding, too hysterical, or even too dumb. It becomes vitally important to be liked by the professional who will be holding your life in his/her hands.

What we tend to forget is that we are not just patients. We are also consumers. As such, we ought to be able to make reasonable requests of our doctors, and have those requests met. In order to accomplish this, we must first identify what our own needs are, and then we must communicate them clearly to our doctors. If this communication is not antagonistic but simply a request for information, there is no reason to assume that it will be met with anger. For example, if you are being scheduled for a mastectomy and all you know about the procedure is that you will awaken without one or both of your breasts, your questions to the doctor might sound like this:

Doctor, in order to feel less fearful, I need more information about this surgery. These are the questions I would like you to answer. How long will the surgery take? Where will the incision begin and end? What kind of scar will I have? What are the risks involved, and how common are those risks? What may I expect immediately after surgery? What kind of pain will I have? How will that pain be managed? How long will I be in the hospital? What is involved in my recovery, and how

long should that take? Do you have a picture to show me of
how I will look after surgery?

This is by no means an exhaustive list. Everyone's concerns are to
some extent unique, and your questions will reflect that. Remember
to take a writing pad, a tape recorder, or a clear-thinking friend with
you so that anything you have trouble retaining is available to you
after your session with the doctor is over.

Many women also fear being thrust into the alien environment
of a hospital, where they have little control over what is done to
them and all the routines and procedures seem ominous because they
are unknown. Questions to ask about the hospital itself might sound
like this:

Doctor, I am very unfamiliar with hospital routines, and I find
that this adds to my fears. Could you or one of your staff tell
me what I can expect? What is the admission process like? What
do I need to bring with me as far as insurance information?
What personal items will I need? Are there things I should not
bring with me? Will there be any other procedures or tests,
besides the surgery, that I will need to undergo while I am in
the hospital? If so, would you explain them to me? Will I receive
any shots or other medication before surgery? How many people will be sharing my room? When are visiting hours? What
time will I go to surgery? How will I get to the operating
room? What is the recovery room like? How long do I have
to wait after surgery before I can go back to my room? What
do I do if I need to speak with you while I'm in the hospital?
Will you visit me in the hospital after surgery is over?

Again, these are only sample questions. You may have no need for
some of them, while others may direct your thinking to areas you
had overlooked before. The process of defining your particular needs
is of crucial importance.

Just a brief word on the value of rehearsal. Can you imagine seeing
a play that had never been rehearsed? Not only would the perfor-

mance be clumsy, but the anxiety level of the actors and actresses would be extremely high. Rehearsal is a way of becoming more familiar with the task at hand, and reducing fear from the level of terror down to nervousness of manageable proportions. Unfortunately, there is no way to rehearse surgery, and a tour of the hospital with introductions to the hospital staff is usually unrealistic. Collecting information is a way of rehearsing and can be a great help in relieving some presurgical anxiety. It is a way of familiarizing yourself with the hospital environment as well as the surgical procedure, so that you don't feel so lost and helpless.

Underlying much of the anguish that women experience as they move through diagnosis and treatment is a feeling of loss of control. There are two things that can help to alleviate this. The first is a shift in attitude from victim to participant. If you perceive surgery as a terrible thing that is being done to you against your will, you are a victim. On the other hand, if you are being offered a procedure that might very well save your life, and you choose it because you greatly value your life, you are a participant. That does not mean that you must look forward to the surgery. It simply puts you in a position of greater control because you have made the choice. The second way to gain control is to have a good rapport with your doctor. For me, having a surgeon who would respond to my questions and inspire my confidence was critical.

The doctor who performed my first surgery was technically excellent. The problem was that our personalities did not seem to mesh well. I felt that it was up to me to put together a health-care team that I could relate to in a more personal way. Shortly after my discharge from the hospital, I began to search for a highly competent surgeon with a good bedside manner and a compassionate approach to his patients. I was fortunate to find Dr. G——, a member of a prestigious surgical oncology group and head of the breast cancer clinic at UCLA Medical Center. When I first met him, I was struck by the genuineness of his concern, the attentive way he listened, and the warmth of his smile. Together we decided that the procedure I had already undergone should be sufficient, and that six weeks of radiation would be the only further treatment needed. At the time, neither of us expected that I would ever need any more surgery, but he agreed to be the overseer of my case, and to see me periodically for checkups. Feeling confident about my choice, I finished a course of radiation and put my concerns about cancer behind me.

Three-and-a-half years later, I had a recurrence. At that point, the only option open to me was a mastectomy. It was a frightening time, but I could always count on Dr. G—— for a kind word and a hug. It took almost two weeks before all the scans were done and I was actually scheduled for surgery.

The night before surgery, I was finally alone in my hospital room when Dr. G—— walked in. It was after ten o'clock, and he had just gotten out of emergency surgery. "Hi," he said. "I was in the neighborhood and thought I would drop by. How are you doing?"

"I am really scared," I replied.

With no regard at all for the lateness of the hour, he sat down on the edge of the bed and asked, "Are you afraid you're going to die?" I shook my head. That didn't feel like my immediate concern. "Well," he continued, "are you worried about what you will look like when your surgery is over?" Once again, I shook my head. Although I was certainly distressed about the impending changes in my body, that did not seem to be the cause of my fear. "Ronnie," he said, "let's take the time right now to figure out what is scaring you." With that, he sat back quietly, as if he had all the time in the world, and gave me an opportunity to do a little searching inside myself.

Suddenly it became very clear. "I know what it is," I said. "I hate the idea that I will be unconscious tomorrow, and people will be doing things to my body without me being present. Having no control frightens me terribly."

"That's exactly what would frighten me, too," he confessed. "But there is a way of solving that. You need to choose someone you trust and turn the control over to him."

"Dr. G——," I responded, "you know how much I trust you. I choose you."

"Fine. Then you can relax. Tomorrow I'll be in charge for both of us." With that, he stood up, gave me a quick hug, and left. Feeling as though someone had lifted a giant mountain off my shoulders, I drifted off to sleep.

chapter five

———————— □ ————————

PHYSICAL RECOVERY
FROM SURGERY

*O*nce surgery is over, a woman who has been diagnosed with breast cancer moves into the next phase of treatment. At the very least, this involves the physical recovery from surgery. In addition, radiation, chemotherapy, hormone therapy, or some combination of these may be required. Many concerns arise during this time relating to physical side effects and the emotional responses to those side effects, and women find themselves, once again, in unfamiliar territory. To allay feelings such as fear, confusion, discouragement, and powerlessness, there is a clear need for information. Women who are well-informed about treatment and also have the opportunity to share and communicate their feelings find that they are much better able to regain a sense of power, mastery, and control.

Limited range of motion in the arm is one of the most common aftereffects of breast cancer surgery. Many women find that they are unable to lift their arm even to shoulder height. This can be very discouraging if no one has prepared you for it in advance. What good will preparation do? If you find that your arm motion is limited, you will already know that there are specific stretching exercises designed to restore full function, and, more important, you will know that the condition is not permanent.

With breast cancer, there are indeed some losses that are permanent. If you lose a breast, you will never have it back again. You may undergo reconstruction, but you will still have lost that original breast. You may also now see yourself as vulnerable. While vulnerability is a fact of life for everyone, we are fairly successful at denying it until we confront a crisis like breast cancer. Then, even though it may seem illogical, we tend to experience the awareness of our own vulnerability as a permanent loss. Because breast cancer makes women particularly sensitive to loss, it is essential that we be able to discriminate between the temporary and the permanent. For permanent losses, we must grieve. For temporary ones, we must find ways of becoming more patient while doing whatever is necessary to deal with the current situation.

Whether the issue is recovering range of motion in the arm, coping with pain following surgery, or with the side effects related to other aspects of treatment, it is vital to understand that everyone is unique, and, depending on the individual, reactions to any treatment can range from none to mild to severe. After my first surgery, I experienced a great deal of pain. It took three days before I was able to get out of bed and attempt a short walk. Slowly and carefully making my way down the hospital corridor, I happened to shuffle past a room filled with brightly colored balloons. There in the bed sat a most beautiful woman, her makeup meticulously applied. She waved at me and invited me in. As I perched gingerly on the edge of the chair, she introduced herself and began to chat.

It turned out that she and I were both breast cancer patients, and had been operated on exactly the same day, just an hour apart, by the same surgeon. Her lymph nodes had been removed just as mine had. I was in considerable pain, and she hadn't taken so much as an aspirin! As we talked, she did something that I considered quite miraculous at the time. She raised both arms and began to tease her hair. I just couldn't understand how she was able to do that. My arm felt as though it had been nailed to my side, and the simplest movement was agonizing. Not having been told how variable individual responses could be, I became deeply depressed and thought that either the surgeon had made a mistake during my surgery or I had a poor attitude and was creating problems for myself. Three years later, I breezed through my second surgery with no pain at all, and was discharged from the hospital after two days. While there really doesn't seem to be any way to account for these differences, the important thing is not to set expectations for yourself based on either your own previous experience or that of others.

But I can offer a word of encouragement as well as one of caution. Doing the stretching exercises is *very* important, and if you discipline yourself to do them regularly, you will probably get your full arm movement back within a relatively short period of time. However, I have noticed a problem that, although by no means typical, has been appearing with some regularity among the women in my groups. They complain of severe pain in their upper arm and/or shoulder, and because they are so anxious to be "good" patients, the worse the pain gets, the harder they exercise. Finally, they are unable to move the arm at all. They experience considerable discomfort and have a real sense of themselves as failures. These women were suffering from either tendinitis (an inflammation of the tendon) or a frozen shoulder, each of which should be treated by an orthopedic surgeon or a physical therapist. Part of the problem was their unwillingness to communicate the difficulty they were having to their surgeon when it first began to occur. Some were reluctant to "bother" the doctor, while others were determined to follow instructions to the letter to prove that they were cooperative patients. A few women had a secret fear that the pain meant cancer had spread into their arm and they just didn't want to hear any more bad news. Others believed that asking for any help at all was admitting defeat and preferred to take charge of the whole process themselves. Whether the issue is fear, embarrassment, or simply a bruised ego, if you find that the exercises are not going smoothly, tell your doctor! While most women can handle the process without help, some need physical therapy for a short period of time in order to regain full range of motion in the arm.

One of the best-kept secrets about breast cancer surgery is the drain that is inserted somewhere near the surgical site. The purpose of this drain is to prevent a painful buildup of fluid in the area. As fluid accumulates, the drain channels it to some receptacle outside the body.

The first time I had surgery, I had a rather strange experience with this drain. I had been wheeled up from the recovery room and was lying in my bed after surgery, only marginally aware that the room was growing darker as the sun was beginning to set. The pain medication I had been given had left me in a semi-doze. I was completely oblivious to the tube that had been inserted in my side during surgery, the other end of which was now connected to a suction pump mounted in the wall behind my bed. However, I was aware that my friend Paula and her husband, Gary, had entered the room. I couldn't seem to get my eyes to focus, and my brain felt pretty foggy, but, for some reason, my sense of hearing remained very acute. I heard Paula's footsteps as she approached my bed. I waited, expecting a sympathetic voice to begin murmuring some reassuring words to me. What I actually heard was a very loud thump, followed by a second set of footsteps, as Gary gasped, "Oh my God!" The next sound was that of a body being dragged across the floor. I don't remember anything after that, having finally succumbed to the effects of the drugs. It wasn't until the next day that I was conscious enough to hear the whole story. It seems that Paula took one look at the drain, saw the blood-tinged fluid moving through it, and immediately passed out. Instead of being affronted at Paula's reaction, I found myself feeling highly flattered that she cared enough about me to have such a spectacular response.

During my recovery, I didn't have to bother with the drain itself. Whenever I needed to get out of bed, a nurse would come and unhook me, until finally I learned to unhook myself. By the time I left the hospital, the doctor had already removed the drain. When I had my second surgery, the setup was very different. I awoke from surgery to find two tubes dangling from my side, each one ending in a kind of bulb. Fluid was draining into each of the bulbs, and wherever I went, so did they. There was something eerie and rather sickening about watching the fluid drain as I walked around. I wanted desperately to get out of the hospital as soon as possible and was discharged in two days, on the condition that I would empty those bulbs religiously twice a day and measure and record the amount of fluid collected. I must admit that it took every ounce of courage I had to agree. I felt surprisingly squeamish, and it was several days before I could handle the task with any measure of self-confidence.

I have spoken to many breast cancer patients since then and have discovered that my reaction was certainly not unique. Given the choice, some women elect to remain in the hospital for a few extra days so that the drain can be removed before they are discharged. If only I had been prepared, I am convinced that much of the shock and revulsion I felt when I was confronted with these hanging drains could have been avoided. I hate surprises when it comes to anything medical. If I had been told in advance about the drain, if it had been described to me in detail, I would have had time to rehearse the management of the situation in my own mind. The more we know, the more prepared we can be, and the better we are able to cope.

Although it is by no means the norm, fluid may sometimes continue to collect near the site of the surgery even after the drain is removed. When this complication occurs, the doctor must be informed immediately. The fluid can be drained in the doctor's office, and the procedure is usually not painful. When the fluid continues to accumulate again and again, women tend to become discouraged and depressed, fearing that the condition is permanent. There are a few things you need to know if you are dealing with this situation. First, be assured that your surgeon has encountered this problem before. Second, you have not done anything wrong, and it is not your fault. And third, no one drains forever. Whether it takes an extra week or more than a month until the draining tapers off, knowing that it is not permanent may help you look on it as a temporary nuisance rather than a life sentence.

Fatigue is another very common aftereffect of surgery. For some reason, once people wake up from surgery, they believe their energy level should return to normal immediately. What they fail to realize is that, although surgery only takes a few hours, the body undergoes a tremendous assault. General anesthesia alone can leave the body tired and drained for a relatively long time. Some of my patients who had surgery as their only treatment for breast cancer have told me that it took many months before they felt that their vitality was fully restored.

Unfortunately, it is sometimes very simple for well-meaning family members, friends, or even a physician to write off fatigue as depression. It is not unusual for a woman who is complaining of exhaustion to be told that she is just depressed. Then, not only is she fatigued, but she also feels guilty for creating her own fatigue by being depressed! The problem is that sometimes it works the other way. Depression can actually be a response to fatigue. Along with other losses sustained as a result of breast cancer, it can be very upsetting and depressing to think that you may also have lost the energetic person you have known yourself to be in the past. Instead of automatically discounting fatigue, or interpreting it as depression, use it as an opportunity to learn to respect the signals your body is sending you. If the message from your body is, "I've been through a lot, and I need time to rest and recover," pay attention. If you want your body to support you, you must take good care of it and attend to its needs. The need for increased rest after surgery makes very good sense. If consistent rest and a slower pace do not make any difference at all in the way you feel, you can then investigate the possibility of depression and its impact on your energy level.

Another problem that may arise as a result of surgery is called **lymphedema**, which is simply a swelling in the arm caused by a collection of excess fluid. This results from damage to or removal of the lymph nodes under the arm. Radiation may also contribute to this condition. When surgery under the arm was more extensive, arm swelling used to occur more frequently. Now it is much less common, but it does happen to some women. Once again, we must look at both the physical condition and the emotional response to it. Sometimes, women feel even worse about a swollen arm than a mastectomy. While one can dress in such a way that the missing breast is not apparent to anyone else, a swollen arm may be more difficult to hide, and can make wearing some clothes awkward. What this amounts to is another loss, and, as with any loss, you can expect to feel angry, resentful, sad, depressed, or any combination of the above. The first thing is to identify your feelings and communicate them. If you find that you need to grieve, do it. If you need to pour out some anger, do that. If the people around you are uncomfortable with your feelings because they can't change the situation, let them know that listening helps and that you don't expect them to do anything else. Don't let anyone make you feel guilty by insisting that you have your life and you shouldn't be worrying about an arm. You will eventually come to terms with your arm, and you will be glad you have your life, but first you need to acknowledge your feelings and have the space to express them.

There are some positive actions to be taken that can help with the physical aspect of lymphedema, the most important of which is to tell your doctor. He/she can prescribe exercises, a specially fitted elastic sleeve or, if necessary, an intermittent compression pump.* In addition, when your arm is not in use, keep it elevated. With your doctor's permission, explore the possibility of massage, which can be extremely helpful in reducing swelling and has become a very popular treatment throughout Europe.

Whether or not you ever experience lymphedema, if your surgery has in any way damaged or removed lymph nodes, there is a chance that your ability to fight infection in the affected arm may be impaired. For that reason, breast cancer patients must take some extra precautions to prevent infection before it starts. Your surgeon should give you a list of do's and don't's—some simple rules to follow that may help you avoid a problem altogether. Some of the common-sense precautions recommended by the National Cancer Institute† include:

* This is an air compressor attached to a special sleeve that is worn over the affected arm. The unit pumps air into the sleeve, maintains a specified level of pressure for a short period of time, and then releases the pressure. This cycle is repeated continuously, creating a pumping action designed to help move the excess fluid out of the arm.

† For more detailed information, a free pamphlet, entitled *After Breast Cancer: A Guide to Followup Care,* may be obtained from the National Cancer Institute by calling the Cancer Information Service at 1-800-4-CANCER.

- Avoid burns while cooking or smoking;
- Have all injections, vaccinations, blood samples, and blood-pressure tests done on the other arm whenever possible;
- Wear protective gloves when gardening and when using strong detergents;
- Avoid harsh chemicals and abrasive compounds;
- Use a thimble when sewing;
- Never cut cuticles; use hand cream or lotion instead;
- Avoid sunburn;
- Use insect repellent to avoid bites and stings;
- Avoid elastic cuffs on blouses and nightgowns, and wear watches or jewelry loosely, if at all, on the treated arm; carry heavy handbags on the other arm;
- Use an electric razor with a narrow head for underarm shaving to reduce the risk of nicks or scratches;
- Wash cuts promptly, treat them with antibacterial medication, and cover them with a sterile dressing; check often for redness, soreness, or other signs of infection.

If, as a result of surgery, a woman has lost one or both of her breasts, she is faced with an obvious difficulty the moment she leaves the hospital. How does she appear in public without feeling awkward, embarrassed, and self-conscious? Initially, the answer is to wear very loose-fitting shirts and tops, and it is important to have one at the hospital so that you can wear it going home. Although you may still feel very conspicuous, it is unlikely that anyone else will notice. A visit from a Reach to Recovery volunteer may be especially valuable at this time. She will bring along a kit containing many helpful items, including a soft cotton puff that can be used as a temporary filling inside a bra cup until a real **breast prosthesis** (artificial breast form) can be purchased. Because your chest may feel quite tender and sensitive for some time, it may be a while before you are comfortable trying on a bra. Check with your doctor to find out exactly what your restrictions are in this regard. When you have his (her) permission, you might want to experiment temporarily with a stretch bra, because they tend to be much more comfortable and less binding. At this point, anything you use as stuffing should be soft and lightweight. Once the skin and underlying tissue at the surgical site are sufficiently healed, your doctor will write a prescription for a prosthesis.

Some women find the idea of being fitted for a prosthesis upsetting. A few of the women I have worked with kept putting it off until they finally realized that they were trying to avoid facing the reality of the loss they had suffered. Others just felt uncomfortable about having to show their surgery to a total stranger. In addition, most women had never seen a prosthesis before and had no idea what they should be looking for. As always, when dealing with the unknown, knowledge helps to restore a feeling of control. There are several ways to see what a prosthesis looks like before you buy one. The American Cancer Society has a display once a month where many different brands and styles are available for inspection. The Society will also provide you with a list of shops in the area that fit prostheses, as well as the brands that each shop carries. It is also valuable to meet with someone who is already comfortable wearing a prosthesis, especially if she is willing to show you how it looks inside her bra. Before selecting a shop, it is wise to ask other women for their recommendations. You may discover that there are some stores that pride themselves on their warm, compassionate, and competent fitters. These are women who tend to be very understanding, and have a wonderful ability to put their customers at ease.

When you are ready to buy your prosthesis, call first and set up an appointment for a fitting. That way, you will be taken into a dressing room immediately, and you won't have to wait around feeling uncomfortable and awkward. Spend a little time chatting with your fitter before you take off your shirt, so that an atmosphere of trust can be established. Ask her how long she has been fitting women for breast prostheses. Most of these women have had years of experience and are knowledgeable as well as kind.

Bring some of your bras with you, because they may be perfectly suitable to hold a prosthesis and you may not need to purchase a special "mastectomy bra." There are some shops that will sew a pocket into your own bra if you feel it necessary. The purpose of the pocket is to hold the prosthesis securely and keep your skin comfortable as well. Many of the stores that sell prostheses also carry a line of swim wear. Women are often amazed and relieved to find that there are many stylish swimsuits that can be easily adapted to accommodate a breast prosthesis. It is also a good idea to bring a close-fitting sweater to try on after you have chosen a prosthesis. When a prosthesis is well fitted, you should look natural, and a sweater is often the best test. If you have had both breasts removed, you do not necessarily need to buy prostheses that match your original size. Some women who had been extremely large-breasted find this a relief, and purchase prostheses in a smaller size, especially enjoying the fact that they are lighter in weight. If you are not satisfied with what you see, say so. There are many different brands, and something else might suit you better. If the shop you have chosen has a limited stock, feel free to look elsewhere. Losing a breast is no reason to give up your right to be an intelligent and selective consumer.

chapter six

RADIATION

*R*adiation therapy, which uses high-energy beams like X rays or gamma rays, destroys cancer cells in a specific area. For that reason, radiation is frequently indicated in the treatment of breast cancer, especially after a lumpectomy has been performed. Exposure is confined to the breast area and, possibly, to the surrounding lymph nodes. For the most part, side effects that accompany radiation treatment depend on the area being radiated. Many of the side effects that people associate with radiation, like nausea and hair loss (from the head), simply do not occur during breast cancer treatment. It is true that hair loss will occur when the head is radiated directly, and nausea and diarrhea are often side effects when the gastrointestinal tract is the target of radiation therapy. However, since the breast lies outside the body cavity and the radiation is aimed at just the superficial area, the internal organs are unlikely to be affected in any significant way, and the head is completely out of range.

As with most other treatments for breast cancer, there are both physical and emotional side effects associated with radiation therapy. Most of the physical ones apply just to the area being radiated: mild to severe "sunburn," itching, tingling, change in skin pigment, change in consistency of the breast tissue (the radiated breast may feel somewhat firmer after radiation), inflammation of the lining of the esophagus, and loss of hair under the arm. With the exception of severe skin burning, usually experienced by women with very fair and sensitive skin, these side effects do not usually cause women any significant physical distress. Even the burns tend to resolve very rapidly after treatment is over.

However, as always, any body changes can trigger an emotional reaction. If you notice changes in skin color, firmness of breast tissue, or breast sensitivity, don't be surprised if you find yourself feeling sad, angry, or even frightened. Give yourself time to express your feelings and to adjust to the changes. Also, be sure to check with your doctor. Most women are advised before treatment that there will be certain changes in the breast area as a result of radiation therapy. It is not unusual, however, for women to feel so overwhelmed and distraught at the time that they have no memory whatsoever of receiving the information. Whether your doctor has informed you or not, a consultation at this time can prove to be very reassuring. You will find that your doctor is familiar with the changes and considers them well within the normal range of responses to radiation. This is another time to bring along your tape recorder so that you can review the information at your leisure.

The physical side effect that many women find the most disturbing is the fatigue that often results from radiation. Not all patients experience this fatigue. Some manage to get through the entire treatment feeling just a little tired toward the end. Others, however, begin experiencing a strange kind of exhaustion after about ten days. It is not the same kind of fatigue that we feel when we have only gotten a few hours of sleep. When that is the case, either a nap or a good night's sleep will handle the problem. If there is a very important task to be accomplished, we can usually muster up enough energy to meet the challenge, even if we are very tired. The fatigue that comes from radiation is different. Many women report that they must either lie down or they will fall down! As treatment progresses, the exhaustion may intensify.

It is quite common to feel deeply distressed about this state of energy depletion. A sudden or progressive loss of energy that severely limits what you are able to accomplish in a day is likely to play havoc with your sense of self. The emotional responses to the situation include depression, despair, anger, impatience, and self-criticism. While these reactions are understandable, they can actually act to magnify the impact of the radiation-induced fatigue. The best thing to do is to speak to someone who has been through radiation and has already recovered her vitality. There is nothing more reassuring than hearing firsthand that this is a temporary state. Although speed of recovery is very individual, most women begin to feel considerably more energetic within a month after radiation ends. This is also a time to appreciate the fact that your body has to work very hard to cope with radiation. Rather than making extra demands on your body at this time, support its efforts to rest and recoup.

A whole complex of feelings that are not based on any physical side effects may also accompany radiation therapy. When women get together and share, these are some of the issues that come up repeatedly: fear of the machines, fear of radiation, and fear of technician error. While not all women experience them, they are fairly common and should be addressed. It is important to select a radiation oncologist who has a good reputation and is experienced with this type of treatment. It also makes very good sense to let the doctor and the technicians know that you are having these concerns. If you say nothing, everyone assumes that you are doing well and that all your needs are being met. Somehow, when you let health-care professionals know that you are fearful, you are treated with a little extra consideration.

Even with reassurance, it can be scary to find yourself lying under a large, strange-looking machine, especially when that machine is the source of radiation—something we of the nuclear-bomb generation have been taught to fear from childhood. There are several things that can prove helpful in this situation. Ask the doctor to explain the **simulation and treatment planning** procedure to you. The purpose of this procedure is to ensure that normal tissue is protected as much as possible. Before you are ever exposed to high-energy radiation, you will go through a process where the dosage and direction of the radioactive beams are carefully computed, checked, and rechecked using low-dose X rays. At that time, the skin in the area to be radiated will be marked with some sort of guidelines. Some doctors use a special marking pen to draw the lines. Because these lines must not be washed off until after treatment is over, women are asked to be very careful when bathing, and showers are out of the question. Other doctors prefer to have a few tiny dots tattooed on the skin. This procedure is painless, but the dots are permanent. The purpose of marking the skin is to enable the technician to align the beam in exactly the same way throughout the entire course of treatment.

Many women find it helpful to be "introduced" to the machine a day or two before treatment actually begins. This can easily be arranged by either the doctor or the technician. You will find that you don't feel nearly as overwhelmed if you are standing on your feet the first time you encounter the machine, rather than lying on the table looking up. Be sure to ask if that particular machine makes any noise during the actual treatment so that if you hear something you won't be alarmed. Finally, there are some patients who have a strong reaction to being left alone during treatment. Old, familiar feelings of abandonment are stirred up, and patients tend to feel very young and unprotected as that lead-lined door slams shut when the technician leaves the room. There is always a two-way communication system connecting the treatment room to the outside. Most technicians will be glad to keep in voice contact with you, if they are told that you would find it helpful. Sometimes a friendly voice asking you how you are doing is enough to relieve some of the fear and the loneliness.

Many of my patients have found "imagery techniques" very helpful in dealing with their anxieties about radiation. While any number of images will work well, it is a good idea to choose one and practice with it for several days before treatment begins. For example, you might imagine yourself lying on the treatment table as a beam of white, healing light emerges from the machine and enters your body. Imagine this light seeking out cancer cells and ridding your body of them. Create as vivid a picture as you can. Once you are actually in the treatment room, re-create that image. Use it every time you receive a treatment. By aligning yourself with the healing process in this way, you will be able to feel less fearful and more in control. The radiation that may have been perceived as a threat can now be transformed into an ally.

If you receive your radiation treatments in a large hospital complex, you are likely to find yourself in a waiting room in the company of other cancer patients. Many women report that this experience was quite grim. I can well remember my first morning at UCLA, waiting for treatment to begin. I was all alone in unfamiliar territory and terribly apprehensive. As I entered the waiting room, I saw couples huddled together, each enveloped in fear and totally isolated from everyone else in the room. Sometimes I could identify the patient, especially the ones who were getting radiation to the brain. They were bald and had "maps" drawn on their heads with purple marking pens. I found that very frightening. But scarier still was the atmosphere that pervaded the room. If there was any talking at all, it was in the softest whisper. When a technician came to the door and called someone's name out, a palpable wave of dread would ripple around the room. During the first three days of my treatment, I spent a total of an hour in that waiting room, oppressed by a terrible sense of isolation and foreboding. By the time I reached the treatment room, I was thoroughly upset.

On the fourth day, I decided to make some changes. I walked into the waiting room and quietly asked, "Is anyone else feeling as scared as I am?" The response was amazing. It was as though someone had opened the floodgates! People introduced themselves and began to talk. In a very short time we had created our own informal support group. The waiting room had become a place where hopes and fears could be shared. We would cheer when a "member" announced the end of treatment, and we would make it our business to welcome newcomers. Together we learned that cancer patients are merely people who happen to have cancer. We learned to see past the disease. Out of a frightening and dangerous environment, we had created a warm haven. It is important to recognize that communicating your own truth can create a wonderful bridge to others and that reaching out is usually worth the risk.

When a woman undergoes radiation therapy following a lumpectomy, it takes approximately five to six weeks for the prescribed amount of radiation to be administered. After that, she will most likely receive what is called a **booster**. This is a dose of radiation directed exclusively to the area where the breast lump was found. This booster may be administered either externally or internally. When the external method is chosen, an electron beam from a type of linear accelerator is aimed specifically at one small area of the breast. Completing the booster dose usually takes five to ten days. I rarely hear complaints about this particular type of treatment other than some skin irritation or redness.

Some physicians still prefer to administer the booster internally, although this method is much less common than it used to be. An internal booster involves the *temporary* implanting of radioactive material in the breast. A hospital stay is mandatory. Upon admission to the hospital, a woman will undergo a minor surgical procedure in which a number of thin plastic tubes are threaded through the breast tissue around the site where the original lump was removed. Either local or general anesthesia is used. Once she returns to her room, radioactive seeds (usually iridium) will be inserted into the tubes, and will remain there for approximately two to three days. At the end of that period of time, the tubes and their contents will be removed, and the patient will be discharged.

I have spoken to many women who have told me how dreadful this experience had been for them. What they were reporting had nothing at all to do with any physical discomfort. While the implant is in place, small amounts of radiation are emitted. For that reason, patients with radioactive implants are put in private rooms, and contact with the nursing staff and visitors must be severely limited. Unfortunately, because many women are not adequately prepared for this experience, they can suffer terribly from fear, loneliness, and isolation. In addition, the idea of being "radioactive" is terrifying! One of my patients told me that she spent her entire hospital stay crying because she thought she would be radioactive forever, and no one would ever be able to hug her again. She had not been told that once the implant is removed, there is no risk to others of radiation exposure. While the implant itself was radioactive, she was not. Another patient recounted her experience with a nurse who spoke to her from the hallway, entered her room reluctantly, and, when her job was done, literally ran. The truth is, because nurses are exposed to this situation frequently, they do need to be concerned about the cumulative amounts of radiation they absorb over a long period of time. Because this had never been explained to my patient in advance, she had felt profoundly lonely and abandoned.

There are certainly ways to alleviate the emotional distress which is sometimes associated with a radioactive implant. Once again, I want to stress the importance of being adequately informed. Make it a rule of thumb never to submit to any medical procedure until you understand it completely, including its psychological and emotional ramifications. Ask very specific questions about the medical and logistical aspects. With respect to the internal booster, once you know clearly what the rules and limitations will be, you can make a special effort to provide yourself, in advance, with those things that will help you structure your time in "solitary" so you can feel more comfortable and secure. Bring good books, tapes, or any handicrafts that may interest you. Ask family and friends to maintain frequent phone contact with you, and, by all means, bring along your teddy bear! With adequate preparation, you might even find that this quiet time in the hospital comes as a welcome relief from the merry-go-round you may have been on during the beginning stages of breast cancer treatment.

chapter seven

CHEMOTHERAPY

*C*hemotherapy is the use of drugs or medications to treat a disease systemically. These chemicals are administered either orally or by injection and circulate throughout the entire body so they can interact with and destroy malignant cells. Aside from the surgical removal of the breast(s), chemotherapy is the treatment breast cancer patients tend to fear most. Because of the profusion of scary stories relating to this mode of treatment, the unwary and uninformed patient is likely to fall prey to a great deal of "chemythology." Many different drugs are used to treat cancer. Some are more likely to cause side effects, like hair loss and nausea, while others are more often associated with minimal side effects. It is also a fact that the range of responses experienced by different individuals to any particular drug is amazingly wide. A medication that might make one patient sick for a week could have virtually no effect on another patient.

Several years ago, I had a unique opportunity to deal with some of my own fears and preconceived notions about chemotherapy. I received a call from Vicki, an acquaintance of mine who had recently been diagnosed with breast cancer. She had just returned from her oncologist's office, where she was informed that she would have to undergo a course of fairly aggressive chemotherapy. She, too, had heard many of the tales about terrible side effects and violent reactions, and she was terrified. While she had many loving and concerned friends, none of them had any firsthand experience with this type of treatment, and they, too, were frightened. Vicki also happened to live alone, and was afraid she might be incapable of helping herself if she became severely ill. I offered to take her to her first treatment, drive her home, and sleep over, just in case anything serious arose. At the time of my mastectomy, my doctors had decided that I was not a candidate for chemotherapy. Although I had counseled many women who had undergone chemotherapy, I had no personal experience to draw on. Not knowing exactly what I was getting into, I was just a bit less apprehensive than Vicki. She had jumped to the conclusion that I was an expert, and as needy as she was, I was reluctant to disappoint her.

During the time that her first treatment was being administered, Vicki and her doctor kept up a lively conversation. I, on the other hand, kept my eyes glued to Vicki's face, waiting for the first trace of some reaction. When nothing unusual happened, I felt both a sense of relief and an urgent need to get her safely home before disaster struck.

At home, she had a light snack and watched a few movies on television, while I waited in painful anticipation of some dreadful reaction. It grew later and later, and Vicki was getting very sleepy. She pointed me to the guest bedroom and went off to bed. I made very sure that the path from my bedroom to hers was clear of all obstacles. I propped her door open so that I could hear the faintest sound. I maintained my vigil for another two hours before finally giving up and going to bed. About half an hour later, just as I had drifted off to sleep, I heard a faint coughing sound coming from down the hall. I must have broken every Olympic record as I flew down that hall toward Vicki's bedroom, only to find her fast asleep. With my heart pounding, I went back to bed and tried to settle down. A short while later, I heard that same cough. Once again, I was out of bed like a shot and down the hall in no time. Vicki was still resting peacefully with no signs of any distress. This went on all night! I was in and out of bed at least eight more times, and each time the only person in distress was me.

The next morning, a bright and cheerful Vicki bounced into my room to ask how I had slept. Feeling totally wrung out, I described my nocturnal adventures, and asked her about that noise I kept hearing. Laughing, she explained that she had a postnasal drip, which often made her cough at night. It had never occurred to her that I might react to it quite the way I did. After watching her eat a hearty breakfast, I returned home. Those first few days, I phoned her frequently to find out whether she had ever suffered any adverse reaction to her first treatment. The answer was always a delighted and emphatic no. And so it went for Vicki throughout the entire six months of chemotherapy. The only complaint she ever had was increasing fatigue as she got closer to the end of her treatments. I learned a lesson from her that has been reconfirmed a hundred times over. No two people are identical, and reactions to the same drugs may vary from individual to individual, and even from treatment to treatment. While it is wise to be informed about possible side effects, try not to base your expectations on what you hear from anyone else. For all the horrifying stories that you might hear, there are also many good ones around—stories about people who have tolerated treatment well and have simply gone on with their lives.

However, there are many women who do have varying degrees of difficulty with chemotherapy. They can experience side effects ranging from mild to severe. Whenever a group of breast cancer patients meets, it is inevitable that there will be a great deal of attention given to concerns about chemotherapy. First, women tend to compare the specific drugs they are being given, and the way those drugs are being administered. It is often upsetting for them to discover that their protocol is different in some significant way from the treatment that other women are receiving. This tends to highlight one of the difficult truths about breast cancer treatment. In many cases, there are several options but no one exclusive right way. If there were a clear-cut answer—a single treatment that always worked—everyone would be using it. It is hard to accept the fact that much of what is being done for breast cancer today lies in a gray zone where a "best guess" based on clinical trials and statistics is the only thing doctors have to guide them. Oncologists use different combinations of drugs, which they may administer in different ways, for many reasons, including: type of cancer, stage of the disease, age of the patient, and the belief that a certain routine may reduce side effects. They must always be concerned about balancing the effectiveness of treatment against the patient's ability to tolerate that treatment.

When it comes to specific side effects of chemotherapy, the ones that seem to cause patients the most physical and emotional distress include nausea, hair loss, depression, and fatigue. Nausea, fatigue, and even depression can be physically debilitating. In addition, the emotional responses to these as well as other chemotherapy side effects cover a very broad range. Women report feeling vulnerable, out of control, fearful, sick, helpless, drained, angry, discouraged, ashamed, hopeless, exhausted, and victimized. Sometimes, a sense of "unwellness" is so pervasive that one of my patients described chemotherapy as "the second illness," the first, of course, being breast cancer. Group support during this period of time is invaluable. Just as important, however, is the constant reassurance I give my patients that the effects are, for the most part, temporary. No matter how comforting patients find that reassurance in the moment, it always seems to bear further repetition. It is hard to attach much reality to the word "temporary" when you are right in the middle of chemotherapy and the months of treatment stretch into the future in a seemingly endless way. Happily, after treatment is over, chemotherapy patients can expect to regain their energy level and sense of physical wellness. Hair will grow back, and any chemically induced mood changes will level off.

The battle to overcome nausea and vomiting should be waged as a cooperative effort with your doctor. He/she will administer or prescribe certain medications to make you as comfortable as possible. What many women don't know is that, if one drug or combination of drugs doesn't work well, there are others to try. It is very important to let your doctor know if you are having a difficult time, so that the necessary adjustments can be made. In addition, many of the women in my groups have found certain nonmedical strategies to be very helpful. These include acupuncture, meditation, stress reduction, guided imagery, mild exercise, and sea bands (wristbands worn by sailors to prevent seasickness), which are available in marine supply stores. A woman's level of stress can have a significant effect on the severity of her reaction to treatment. There have been many times when a patient has come to a group session to share that her most recent treatment had been unusually difficult. We would review the past few weeks and often find that her stress level had been uncommonly high. After taking whatever steps are necessary to reduce the stress in her life, she is likely to report that her next treatment was markedly better, with fewer severe side effects. It also helps to communicate with other women who are facing the same problem. Just knowing you are not alone can be comforting, reassuring, and very supportive. In addition, it is extremely valuable to speak with a woman who has already "graduated" from treatment. It serves as an important reminder that chemotherapy is not forever, and people do make it through.

I often find hypnosis and imagery to be very effective with those patients who are having an especially difficult time with chemotherapy. Terri, for example, was a thirty-six-year-old breast cancer patient who came to a group complaining of persistent nausea and unrelenting flulike symptoms, including severe pain in her muscles and joints. She just didn't seem to be able to get comfortable and had mentioned that she would probably be much happier if she could somehow escape from her body for the duration of treatment. With the use of hypnosis, I was able to structure an experience for her which accomplished exactly that!

First, I taught her to relax her body by using deep breathing and focusing on one set of muscles at a time. Once she had moved into a more relaxed state, I invited her to imagine a perfectly safe and very lovely place—a place where she could spend some time in beautiful surroundings while feeling very protected. Once Terri had a clear picture of her retreat, I asked her to find a special place for herself within that picture, and to make sure that she was absolutely comfortable there. Then I suggested that, since she was completely safe and secure in this environment, she could leave her body there without any concerns about it, while she herself could be free to travel anywhere she chose. Without a moment's hesitation, Terri imagined herself leaping from her body, landing gently on an air current, and beginning to fly. I sat by quietly, giving her the space to become fully absorbed in the experience. Later Terri told me that as she traveled around the world she found she could move through the seasons as well. From her vantage point in the sky, she was able to enjoy some truly spectacular aerial views! After a while, I asked her to let me know when she was ready to come back to earth, reassuring her that she would be able to fly again whenever she wished to.

Once Terri signaled that she was willing to stop traveling, I asked her to return to her special place and move into her body once again. The suggestion I left her with was that, simply by using some deep breathing and relaxation techniques, she would be able to return to that special place at will, leave her body behind whenever she needed to, and feel the same freedom that she had experienced this first time. I also suggested that the more she practiced, the more proficient she would become. As Terri emerged from her trance, she remarked on how relaxed and comfortable she felt. Together we reviewed what had happened, and I reminded her again that practice would make this technique even more available to her. Several weeks later, Terri told me that she had mastered the routine so well that she could go from considerable discomfort to free flight within seconds! To the uninitiated, this may sound contrived. However, those people who have had some practice in using imagery will attest to the fact that they become totally absorbed in the images and experience them in an immediate and profound way internally, even though the outer reality does not change.

Another side effect that is especially difficult for most women is **alopecia**, or hair loss. Hair loss occurs because the drugs used in chemotherapy are absorbed mostly by cells that divide rapidly. While cancer cells fall into that category, unfortunately so do some of the normal cells in the body. Other rapidly dividing cells include those in the bone marrow, the gastrointestinal tract, the reproductive system, and the hair follicles. Although they are vulnerable to the effects of anticancer drugs, these normal cells do have a tremendous capacity to regenerate themselves. That means that hair loss is temporary.

Hair will grow back, and sometimes begins to do so even before treatment is over. The question is, what do women do, and how do they feel in the meantime?

Sometimes it is hard for other people to appreciate how devastating hair loss can be for the woman undergoing chemotherapy. Historically, hair has been associated with beauty and femininity just as the breast has been. Some of my patients have told me that losing a breast was much easier than losing their hair. This can be a time when looking in the mirror becomes an ordeal. Every time you see your reflection, you are reminded that something precious, something closely connected with your identity, has been snatched away. Going out in public can be terribly stressful as well. It is hard to believe that you are acceptable to others at a time when your appearance causes you such anguish. Patients have told me that they have felt ashamed, ugly, depressed, angry, unfeminine, sad, vulnerable, and more naked than when they had their clothes off. Because hair loss is so visible, at least to the woman herself, she is confronted constantly with the fact that she is engaged in a battle against cancer.

As with everything else relating to cancer, the first thing to do is acknowledge your feelings. It helps to have people who will listen to you. If they have gone through something similar, that's even better. While meeting and talking with a woman whose hair has already grown back won't change your reality, it lets you know in very concrete terms that this indignity is survivable and temporary. In addition, women tend to pass along helpful hints to each other. One of the things I hear about fairly frequently from women who have lost their hair is the agony of the "fallout" period. I have received frantic phone calls from patients who had been unsuspectingly showering, only to end up with clumps of hair all over the bathroom floor. Some women wake up in the morning and find the pillow literally covered with hair. It is both shocking and frightening when that begins to happen. The best advice from veterans of "fallout" is to waste no time in getting the shortest haircut possible, or, better yet, to have your head shaved completely. This eliminates the daily torment of wondering how much hair you will lose today and how you will look tomorrow. Many women will prepare for hair loss by buying a wig in advance, so that they can get a stylist to match their natural hair as closely as possible. The American Cancer Society has designed a program called "Look Good, Feel Better," which is made available to cancer patients who must cope with hair loss resulting from treatment.

Some women get very creative with hats, scarves, and turbans, turning their inventiveness into fashion statements. Several years ago, I met a unique woman who was going through chemotherapy and had decided to be exactly who she was—a sexy, attractive, bald female. She wore exotic earrings, wild clothes, a lot of blue eye shadow, and no head covering whatsoever. While people may have been shocked initially, in a very short time they found themselves admiring her for her honesty, spunk, and incredible sense of self. Whether you cover up or go "natural," use this opportunity to learn that you are not your hair. You are capable of living, loving, experiencing joy, communicating, and being taken seriously even if you have no hair. The person that you really are, that essence that defines you as a human being, is far more important and valuable than any hairdo.

What about depression? Isn't it fair to say that being confronted with cancer in the first place and then undergoing treatment for it justifies any feelings of depression? Well, yes and no. When it comes to chemotherapy, what many women do not know is that the drugs themselves can induce a depression. Unfortunately, some doctors don't make that information available to their patients. As a result, I get phone calls from women who are terribly troubled because the depression they are feeling seems so much larger, blacker, heavier, and more pervasive than anything they have ever felt before.

I once received a phone call from a woman who told me she felt so horribly depressed and so unlike herself that she was beginning to consider death as a viable alternative. She had always known herself to be a very positive and joyful person, and this radical change was not only frightening but totally unacceptable. When I asked whether she was undergoing chemotherapy, she told me she had received her first treatment just three days before. I asked whether

her doctor had told her about the chemically induced depression that many women experience, which lasts somewhere between three and six days after a treatment. There was a long silence, and then she said, "Do you mean that it's not me after all? It's just the chemicals that are doing this?" She was greatly relieved, but she would have been spared a great deal of distress if she had been warned in advance of this particular side effect. I reassured her as best I could, and asked her to call back within the next few days to let me know how she was doing. The next time she called, it was like talking to a different person. She had begun to feel better the moment she knew where her depression was coming from, and two days after our first conversation it had lifted completely.

Many of the women who have been through my support groups tell me that there is a qualitative difference between the depression caused by chemotherapy and the depression that results from grappling with a crisis like breast cancer. If they really pay attention, they are able to distinguish between the two. Once they can tell the difference, they are in a much better position to deal effectively with their emotions. If the depression is chemical, they simply remind themselves that it will pass, and they try to be as nice to themselves as they can in the interim. On the other hand, if the depression is situational, they make every effort to identify the issues which are distressing them so that they can be dealt with.

Fatigue is another one of the side effects commonly experienced by women who undergo chemotherapy. Some feel their energy level to be only slightly depleted. Others describe this fatigue as an exhaustion so profound that they feel as though they are teetering at the brink of a black hole that periodically swallows them up. For some reason, it seems difficult for people to accept the fact that the body is entitled to feel fatigued when dealing with chemotherapy. These drugs are toxic to cancer cells, which is why they are administered. However, they also present an enormous challenge to the body, which must process and then eliminate them and, at the same time, repair any damage sustained by healthy tissue. Often women find that they simply cannot keep up the same pace they are normally accustomed to.

The emotional reactions to fatigue have already been discussed in the section on radiation, and they are identical in the case of chemotherapy. This fatigue forces a woman to make compromises in the way she plans her day and in the things she is able to accomplish. Some women become depressed about this, others get angry, but many blame themselves and take themselves to task for doing a less-than-perfect job either at work, at home, or both. This is a time to acknowledge that your body has a wisdom of its own. Listen to its signals and respect them. Give yourself permission to put your own needs before the needs of others. Learn to make your recovery your first priority. Instead of equating rest with capitulation or defeat, think of it as one of the gifts you can give your body so that it can continue to participate in the treatment as fully and effectively as possible.

The next complex of side effects which some women complain of includes dizziness, blurred vision, a marked change in near or far vision, an inability to concentrate for extended periods of time, and an impairment of short-term memory. In and of themselves, these can be disturbing because women feel their physical and mental competence is being eroded. When patients are not informed that these can be side effects of treatment, they sometimes come to alarming conclusions. Having somehow learned that breast cancer, when it spreads, can metastasize to the brain, they assume that these particular symptoms are being caused by a brain tumor. Trying to protect themselves against more bad news, they resist sharing their concerns with their doctor. As a result, they go around for weeks or months feeling terrified, just waiting for disaster. I have often seen a look of profound relief on the face of a group member who has just been told that these particular side effects are directly related to chemotherapy and are most definitely temporary.

It is not unusual for sleep disturbances to accompany chemotherapy. Many women have told me that for several days after their treatment, even when they know they are exhausted, they are unable to sleep. The moment they get into bed they seem to be filled with a strange kind of agitated energy. Others say that their whole sleep pattern has been disrupted regardless of where they are in the treatment cycle. The more a patient is deprived of sleep, the more exhausted she becomes. As this exhaustion intensifies, not only does she begin to feel unwell, but her ability to cope with stress, or even with life in general, is greatly reduced. Lack of sleep can be very debilitating, especially at this time. Although I am not usually an advocate of pills, it makes good sense to consult with the doctor who can prescribe some sleep medication when it is appropriate. Even if a woman takes one dose every four or five days, one good night's sleep can be an amazing restorative.

In addition, there are deep relaxation techniques that are simple to learn and provide another way to rest the body (see Supplement). Twenty minutes of deep relaxation can often be the equivalent of a few hours of regular sleep. Relaxation, meditation, and sleep-induction tapes are sold in New Age bookstores and many record shops. If tapes are not available in your area,* the self-help section of your local bookshop will have books on relaxation and self-healing. One of the finest of these is *Healing Yourself* by Martin L. Rossman, M.D. Often these books have scripts you can record to create your own relaxation tapes.

Chemotherapy can have considerable impact on the hormonal balance of the body, causing a myriad of symptoms, among which are mild to severe hot flashes, vaginal dryness, and, for the premenopausal patient, a cessation of the menses. For the younger woman, any interruption in the menstrual cycle will probably be temporary. However, a woman who is closer to the age where menopause would be more likely to occur naturally may experience a sudden and premature onset of menopause. As with most other side effects of breast cancer treatment, there can be both physical and emotional responses to the hormonal effects of chemotherapy.

Some women report a high level of distress with regard to severe and frequent hot flashes. They experience considerable discomfort

---

* For an extensive selection of audiotapes and videotapes, write for a cassette list from The Bodhi Tree Bookstore, 8585 Melrose Avenue, Los Angeles, CA 90069, 213-659-1733. You may request specific categories such as meditation, relaxation, self-hypnosis, healing, or managing the side effects of chemotherapy.

during the day and find that their sleep is completely disrupted by night sweats. Because hot flashes usually accompany a normal menopause, it is sometimes hard for women to get their doctors to take these symptoms seriously. One of my group members, a sixty-six-year-old woman, was having an extremely difficult time with hot flashes. She would perspire so profusely that she had to change her clothes several times a day. She had begun to limit her excursions to the neighborhood market, embarrassed to be caught in public in the middle of one of her hot flashes. Her night sweats were so severe that lack of sleep had become a major problem. She tried telling her doctor that she really needed some help, but because she was so accustomed to taking care of others and so reluctant to burden the busy man, she mentioned it without communicating any sense of urgency. He asked how many episodes she was having in the space of twenty-four hours. Unprepared for the question, my patient was unable to come up with a specific number. Making light of the issue, the doctor told her to get back to him when the hot flashes numbered one hundred a day.

Upset and disheartened, she returned to tell the story to the group. The other members were outraged. Having her difficulties discounted in that manner was absolutely unacceptable! We helped her find ways to communicate her needs and expectations clearly to the doctor so that he would work with her to obtain some relief. In a fairly short period of time, she and her doctor had found a medication which, although it did not eliminate the hot flashes altogether, did bring them down to a tolerable level.

A chemically induced menopause occurs quite suddenly and its symptoms can be more severe than those which accompany a gradually progressing natural menopause. Aside from hot flashes and vaginal dryness, the list of symptoms can include dizziness, heart palpitations, muscle and joint pains, headaches, and sleep disturbances. Normally, a woman going through a difficult menopause is a candidate for hormone replacement therapy. This mode of treatment is usually not made available to the breast cancer patient. Therefore, it is especially important to know that the same nonmedical techniques that work for nausea also have beneficial results in the treatment of hot flashes and many other symptoms of menopause. I consistently recommend that my patients employ some combination of acupuncture, deep relaxation, stress reduction, and mild exercise. I am sometimes amazed at how effective these methods can be. By embarking on a rigorous program of stress reduction and deep relaxation techniques, one of my patients was able to reduce the severity of her symptoms, including hot flashes, from debilitating to mildly annoying within a week.

Being thrown into premature menopause can create emotional as well as physical consequences. Some women are not yet ready to give up the option of having children and feel this loss severely. When a woman has been looking forward to bearing a child, she may feel depressed, sad, deeply disappointed, angry, and resentful should chemotherapy rob her of the opportunity. It is not only the effects of chemotherapy that can impose such a limitation on a woman. A breast cancer diagnosis alone may have serious consequences as far as the appropriateness of a future pregnancy. Some physicians discourage any thought of future pregnancy for the breast cancer patient. Others try to evaluate each case individually.

So far, there is no evidence that pregnancy increases the risk of recurrence. If treatment is completely successful and all cancer cells have been eliminated from the body, recurrence is not an issue. Unfortunately, because individual cancer cells are too small to detect, no guarantee can be offered to a woman who has been treated for breast cancer that she is now completely cancer-free. If there is a chance of recurrence, the radical hormonal shifts that occur during pregnancy may hasten the event. A woman who is highly motivated to undergo a pregnancy after breast cancer has a difficult choice to make. On the one hand, there is an intense longing to bear a child. On the other hand, there are some grave concerns about her responsibility to that child as well as questions about her own longevity. In cases where pregnancy might be feasible, doctors may suggest that a woman postpone it for two to five years.

People experience the disruption of major life plans as a significant loss. They tend to feel helpless and disoriented and need a chance to recover. As always, an opportunity to acknowledge and express feelings is extremely helpful, and expressions of grief are certainly appropriate. Usually a woman will come to terms with the loss of her ability to bear children, recognizing the fact that her life is important and should not be jeopardized. However, if the breast cancer patient blames herself for the loss and feels seriously diminished by it, or if the situation creates a rift between the woman and her spouse, some counseling is advisable. With or without help, this setback must be transformed into a challenge. Not only must a woman come to terms with the loss, but she must also find other ways to put meaning and fulfillment into her life.

Many women approach chemotherapy as a punishment, and each trip to the doctor's office becomes an ordeal. Even though some patients have a difficult time during treatment, it helps to focus on what those chemicals are doing *for* you, rather than what they are doing *to* you. As with radiation, imagery can be a real asset in dealing with chemotherapy. The images my patients have used have been varied and quite creative. One woman imagined the drugs entering her body and being transformed into an army of white knights riding white chargers and armed with lances. The knights used their lances to hunt out and spear cancer cells, rendering them helpless. Several other patients borrowed the idea of "scrubbing bubbles" from one of the commercials on television. In their mind's eye, they saw millions of these bubbles making their way through the body, systematically foaming the cancer cells away. Another woman said that as her treatment was being administered, she pictured the fluid from the syringe dividing up into tiny molecules of light, each of which was extraordinarily powerful. As these molecules circulated throughout her entire body, they used their light to seek out cancer cells. So strong and pure was this light that when it came into contact with a cancer cell, that cell was simply vaporized. No matter what the image, patients who use them report that they feel more hopeful and confident, and much less out of control, because they are actively participating in their own treatment.

Many women deeply resent the fact that the side effects of chemotherapy can be so distressing. They feel that a cancer diagnosis is burdensome enough, and that treatment should therefore be easy.

These feelings are normal and certainly understandable. At times like this, it is especially difficult to come to terms with the fact that not everything in life is easy or fair. Chemotherapy must be thought of as a short-term investment for a long-term gain. Even though side effects may cause considerable discomfort, the whole purpose of the treatment is to control cancer and extend life. When you consciously choose to be in treatment, you can relinquish the role of victim and reaffirm your investment in life.

□

HORMONE
THERAPY

*W*hen a breast lump is first removed for biopsy, a hormone receptor test is performed on the tissue. This test can determine whether a particular cancer is sensitive to the presence of estrogen or progesterone, hormones that are produced normally by the body. A positive result indicates that the cancer will grow in the presence of a particular hormone and will die without it. In these cases, hormone therapy is often indicated. The whole purpose of hormone therapy is to manipulate the hormonal environment inside the body so that cancer cells are prevented from thriving. Sometimes the ovaries are surgically removed, but more often a medication is prescribed that achieves the same result.

The drug most frequently used in hormone therapy for breast cancer is tamoxifen (Nolvadex). Tamoxifen actually prevents estrogen from getting inside cancer cells. This estrogen-blocking property also has an effect on the normal cells of the body. As a result, the body may experience a state of estrogen deprivation. Many women are not affected at all by this type of treatment. However, those who experience some degree of discomfort cite hot flashes, fatigue, and depression as the primary side effects. Symptoms that appear with less frequency may include fluid retention, headache, vaginal discharge, dizziness, menstrual irregularities, nausea, and a distaste for

food. Because many of these symptoms are similar to the ones discussed in the section on chemotherapy, the same kinds of approaches,
both medical and nonmedical, often prove quite effective in alle-
viating them.

Most women seem to fare quite well with tamoxifen. As a general
rule, any side effects tend to diminish and finally disappear over a
period of time. There are some instances, however, when a woman
truly cannot tolerate this medication. Rita was a patient who had
been a very vital, lively, politically active woman her entire life. At
the age of seventy-six, she was operated on for breast cancer. Following surgery, she was put on tamoxifen, and within two months
had lost her appetite, dropped fifteen pounds, and become so fatigued
that a walk around the block would exhaust her for an entire day.
For a while, she struggled to maintain a good front, making light
of her situation. As her symptoms worsened, she became extremely
depressed. The longer the depression continued, the more Rita convinced herself that her emotions were at the root of her physical
distress. She had always been respected for her sharp mind and dynamic approach to life, and she now felt as though people were
thinking of her as a "crazy old lady."

One day, she was looking through her calendar, hoping to find
some event that might have been significant enough to trigger this
terrible depression. She happened to notice that her lack of interest
in food had begun shortly after she had started on tamoxifen. In
desperation, she called her pharmacist and asked him to read the
package insert from her medication. Two of the side effects he mentioned were anorexia (loss of appetite) and fatigue. Once she knew
it wasn't her fault, she called her doctor and told him that she had
lost a lot of weight and was so exhausted she could barely function.
He immediately took her off the tamoxifen. Within a few weeks she
had regained most of her vitality and was enjoying three hearty meals
a day. At that point, her doctor started her on Megace, another drug
used in hormone therapy. Rita has continued to do well and has
experienced no serious side effects from the new drug.

It is rare that a woman will have such a violent reaction to tamoxifen. The complaints that I hear in my groups relating to hormone

therapy have much more to do with lack of information than actual physical discomfort. Women can be sensitive to even the smallest changes in their physical or emotional states. They tend to become anxious and fearful when these changes occur unexpectedly, especially following a cancer diagnosis. It is very reassuring for them to learn that others who are receiving the same treatment may be experiencing similar changes.

Although Rita's story is extreme, there are several important lessons to be learned from it. First, never assume that you are creating your own symptoms. As with all drugs, whether they pertain to cancer treatment or not, a patient can have any reaction at any time. Second, open and ongoing communication with your doctor is a must. Be sure to ask about any *changes* you might detect, rather than limiting your inquiry to symptoms and side effects. Finally, make it your business to be as well-informed as possible, whether by reading, talking with your doctor, meeting with women who are "graduates" of breast cancer treatment, or comparing notes with others who are presently undergoing similar treatment. Knowledge really is power, and being well-informed is one of the very best ways of ensuring your own well-being.

chapter nine

BODY
IMAGE

*i*t was just an ordinary Wednesday night at American Cancer Society headquarters. I was leading the second session of one of my eight-week breast cancer support groups. All twelve participants were recovering from recent surgery, and many were still in active treatment. In order to give the evening a focus and help facilitate some sharing, I will often start the evening off by asking a question. That night, the question was, "What has changed in your life as a result of having had breast cancer?"

As we went around the circle, each woman tried to explain how breast cancer had affected her life. One felt that her friends were now treating her differently, another noticed a serious loss of self-confidence, and a third was experiencing a surprising indifference to future plans. Then it was Gladys's turn. "Going to the gym isn't the same anymore," she said sadly.

As I pressed for more details, she explained, "I'm sixty years old. I used to go to the gym three times a week. Even though I didn't have the most terrific body in the world, I still felt free to run around the locker room without any clothes on. I would go into the Jacuzzi and the steam room naked like everyone else and never think twice about it. Since my mastectomy, it's different. Now I find a locker in a remote corner, undress quickly with my back to everyone, and wrap myself in three towels. One towel goes around my waist, the next one I tie around my chest, and the third I drape around my neck as a kind of insurance, just in case the middle one happens to fall off. I try to sneak into the Jacuzzi when no one else is there. I have even devised a system for removing my towels one at a time. By the time I'm completely out of my towels, I'm under water and no one can see me. I get out the same way, wrapping up one section at a time, so that I'm never exposed. I never take my towels off in the steam room either. I don't feel happy and free anymore when I go to the gym. I just feel different and ashamed."

My response startled the entire group. Everyone was expecting me to get into a deep discussion about body image and loss. Instead, I asked Gladys which gym she attended. As luck would have it, I was a member of the same health club. "Gladys," I proposed, "if you're free on Monday night, let's meet at the gym. We'll go into the locker room together. You can wear your towels, and I'll go bare. The only thing you must agree to do is to make a full report to the group when we reconvene next week." Caught off guard, but willing to risk an adventure, Gladys agreed.

That Monday night, I arrived at the gym, duffel bag in hand, wearing my workout clothes. I had hopes of taking advantage of the evening by squeezing an aerobics class into my busy schedule. Gladys was waiting for me at the door. When I suggested a class, she looked at me as though I might be crazy, grabbed my hand, and dragged me off to the locker room. Clearly, there was another order of business here that took priority!

In the locker room, Gladys took me over to the locker she had found where she had the most protection from exposure. Turning to face the wall, she began to undress. I threw my duffel bag down on a bench, and began to strip off my clothes. Behind me, I heard Gladys's shocked voice, as she began a running commentary. "Oh my God," she whispered. "You're really doing it! I was sure you would back down when we actually got here. Watch out! Someone is coming this way. She may see you. How can you just stand there? How come she didn't even look? Uh-oh, here comes someone else. Maybe you should grab a few towels, just in case. I don't understand

. . . no one seems to be looking at you. Are you sure you don't want a towel?"

Once Gladys was ready, we made our way to the Jacuzzi. She was wrapped in her many towels, and I was nude. My heart went out to her as she inched her way into the Jacuzzi, careful that no part of her chest was ever visible. There were a few other women there, but no one seemed to notice my mastectomy except Gladys, who became more and more nervous with each passing moment. When we were ready to leave the Jacuzzi, Gladys went through the reverse procedure, wrapping herself up again, one towel at a time, until she was completely covered.

She invited me into the steam room with her, but I told her that I preferred the sauna. I asked her to come and get me in ten minutes. Once in the sauna, I began to worry. If no one had a visible reaction to my mastectomy, Gladys would return to the group with very little to report. I decided to stir up a bit of excitement by interviewing the other women in the sauna. I approached one young woman and said politely, "May I ask you a question?" She nodded. "How do you feel about the fact that I have only one breast?" She looked a bit startled. After all, that is not exactly something one would expect to hear in a sauna. "You know," she said, somewhat surprised, "I hadn't even noticed. Now that you call it to my attention, it doesn't seem like a very big deal."

I moved on to the next person. "Pardon me," I said. "Would you tell me what your reaction is to the fact that I am one-breasted?" She answered, "I feel very sorry for you." This time, I was the one who was surprised, since I don't feel sorry for myself at all. When I asked her to explain, she continued, "If you had become macrobiotic, you would never have lost your breast!" I told her that I was referring specifically to my physical appearance, and wondered if she had any particular feelings about that. "Oh no," she replied. "I'm a physical therapist. I'm quite used to seeing this type of thing, and it doesn't bother me at all."

I was still trying to figure out how to turn this into a worthwhile experience for Gladys, when she appeared in the sauna. I introduced her to the women I had already interviewed, hoping that their acceptance of me would have some impact on her. As we left, the first young woman followed us out into the dressing room. Gladys, still wrapped in her towels, parked herself under a hair drier, while the young woman and I, both totally nude, began to chat. It seemed that she had become involved in the real estate business, and wondered if I would be interested in investing in some commercial property. As it happens, the dressing room is situated between the gym and the locker room, and people are passing through constantly. Every few minutes, another woman would stop by and join the conversation. Within a short time, I found myself in the middle of a crowd of women, all of whom were involved in a heated discussion about the advantages and disadvantages of various types of investments, while Gladys watched from the sidelines. After about fifteen minutes, I looked over and saw her standing there with a big grin on her face. Her perception of herself as an outcast had been challenged. She understood that her own lack of self-acceptance and her fear of rejection had made it impossible for her to relax and enjoy her time at the gym. When she actually observed how comfortable I felt about myself and how well accepted I was by others, she was able to let her towels drop to the floor and came over to join the crowd.

When the group met the following week, everyone was eager to hear Gladys's story. She related the whole experience and told the other women how liberated she had been feeling ever since our evening in the gym. The other women were applauding her triumph, when suddenly one of them asked, "What would you have done if someone at the gym had looked at you and then turned away in disgust." The room grew very quiet, as everyone waited for my reply. "No problem," I answered. "I would approach her and say, 'I saw you look at me and then turn away. I was wondering whether you were worried that you would make me feel self-conscious, or whether you had never seen a mastectomy before and felt a bit upset.' I would use the opportunity to educate her. It would never occur to me that the problem was mine." I looked around the room and saw the group members nodding their heads and smiling. Even though their self-confidence had not yet reached that level, they were beginning to see it as a possibility for themselves.

Because I considered the story of Gladys and her adventures in the gym so valuable, I told it to every breast cancer group I led for the next two years. Then, much to my delight, I discovered that the story had a most heartwarming sequel. One evening, outside the Cancer Society headquarters, I ran into Gladys looking radiant and very chic. She had come to attend a Smokenders meeting. I asked her whether she was still going to the same gym.

"Oh yes," she replied, "and since you were always telling us stories, I have one to tell you. Just a few weeks ago, I was walking through the locker room, stark naked, when I was approached by a woman who was all wrapped up in towels. Very hesitantly, she asked, 'Do you know someone by the name of Ronnie Kaye?' When I said that I did, she continued, 'Are you the woman she told us about? Did she really go to the gym with you? Did you actually take off your towels that night?' Smiling, I assured her that the whole story was absolutely true. 'Oh,' she confided, 'I admire you so much. I still can't bring myself to take off any of my towels. I feel frightened and self-conscious, and I don't know if I will ever feel differently.' I was really touched. As I looked at her, I saw myself two years ago, and appreciated how far I have come since then. Putting my arm gently around her shoulders, I said, 'Come with me and I will do for you what Ronnie did for me.' "

Not every breast cancer patient struggles with the issue of body image. Some women never considered their breasts very important, and others feel relieved to have a breast removed if it was a threat to their health and well-being. There are also some women who are so secure in their self-image that the absence of one or both breasts doesn't seem to shake them. However, these women are in the minority. After all, we live in a very breast-centered society. We are taught from the time we are children that breasts are beautiful and sexy and that we must have them if we are to be considered desirable. As girls mature, especially in the early and middle teenage years, those with small breasts are often teased and ridiculed. On the other hand, those girls who develop voluptuous breasts at a fairly early age are often the focus of much admiration and interest from their male counterparts, and may even be the secret envy of their girlfriends. Small-breasted teenagers often wind up feeling inferior.

Many of their well-developed classmates report having felt terribly conspicuous and self-conscious to have been the object of so much attention solely because of their breasts. Regardless of our early experiences, most of us do come to the conclusion that having two breasts is what entitles us to membership in the sorority of adult women, and it is also what makes us desirable to others. Without those breasts, we tend to feel completely unacceptable.

How, then, does a woman recover emotionally when her breast(s) has been marred or removed? As Gladys's story illustrates, there are two separate issues that must be considered. The first is how a woman feels about herself, and the second is her fear of being unacceptable to others. In terms of self-image, the single most helpful experience is to have close contact with a woman who has undergone breast cancer surgery and has reached the point where she has very positive feelings about her own body. I often hear a woman who has just lost a breast say that she can no longer think of herself as whole. The phrase "half a woman" comes up again and again in many of my groups. It is often a revelation for these women to discover that there are many of us in the world who feel attractive, sexy, and secure even though we are missing one or both breasts.

I routinely remove my shirt and show my mastectomy to women who are struggling with body image. The results are often astounding. Jennie, a woman in her mid-sixties, was referred to me by her surgeon. She had undergone a mastectomy six weeks before, and had been unable to look at herself since then. She had gone to great pains to avoid confronting the change in her own body. She bathed with her eyes closed, and whenever she undressed she would drape a towel over her shoulder to hide the surgical site from view. Fear and shame seemed to permeate every waking moment of her day. The first time she came to my office, Jennie was terribly anxious, knowing that she somehow needed to make peace with her body and yet terrified of what that might entail. We chatted for a while, as I took a detailed history. Then I asked her if she had ever seen a mastectomy before. When she said she hadn't, I asked if she had some image in her mind as to what it might look like. "A huge, horrible, angry red wound," she answered, "on a chest that looks as though it has been gouged out. It must look very raw and very ugly." Mastectomies do not look like that at all, but this is a fairly common image held by people unfamiliar with the surgery. Poor Jennie! No wonder she was so frightened. I explained that a mastectomy basically looks like a preadolescent chest without a nipple, and that the surgery is very neat and clean. I offered to show her my scar, but she adamantly refused, saying she just wasn't ready.

As we continued the session, she kept talking about how ashamed and different she felt, and how her feelings were coloring her life. Finally, I repeated my offer. This time, Jennie asked plaintively, "Do I really have to do this?" "No, Jennie, you don't," I said with conviction. "It's just that this is the quickest and most painless way to move you past where you are stuck right now. You will get to look at a mastectomy without looking at yourself. It will give you the opportunity to get accustomed to the appearance of a one-breasted woman." Her face white, her voice small and forlorn, her eyes swimming with tears, she asked, "Will it make me cry?" I could see her inner child at that moment, young, frightened, and vulnerable, and I felt very protective toward her. "It will probably make you cry," I answered, "but you are sitting in a therapist's office, dealing with a serious loss. Crying is very appropriate and it is safe to do it here." She nodded her head and then watched, tears slowly trickling down her face, as I unbuttoned my blouse.

First, I showed her what a bra looks like with a prosthesis inside. Next, I removed the prosthesis and let her hold it in her hand. Her only comment was that it felt surprisingly soft and warm. Then I unhooked my bra and showed her my mastectomy. The office was very quiet. Jennie looked, turned away, and then looked again. Finally, she said, "Well, it's different, but it's not ugly." I invited her to touch the skin on my chest and inspect my scar, which was barely visible. In a short time she had become quite comfortable with my appearance and was able to relax. She told me that she felt as though she had achieved an important victory, and I agreed. When the session was over, I escorted her to the waiting room, where her husband was patiently reading a magazine. He looked up at Jennie, his eyes filled with concern. Jennie grinned as she said excitedly, "Honey, wait until I tell you what we did!"

The following week, Jennie returned for her next appointment.

She was elegantly dressed, which is always a good sign. "I drove here by myself!" she announced proudly. Since her surgery, she had felt so depressed and overwhelmed that she hadn't found the courage or the energy to go anywhere on her own. Her husband had driven her wherever she needed to go. Since our session Jennie had begun feeling much more independent and self-sufficient, which was another good sign. When I asked her how she was doing with her body-image problem, she replied, "I'm not there yet, but I'm on my way. I haven't been able to really look at myself this week, but . . . I peeked!" I assured her that she did not have to adapt herself to any other time schedule than the one that felt right to her. It was obvious that she really was on the way. Within a few weeks, Jennie was able to stop hiding from herself and from her husband. She put to rest many preconceived notions and old stereotypes as she came to understand that she was a valuable and important human being and could not be defined in any way by the presence or absence of a breast.

There may come a point where no matter how much outside support a woman receives, or how powerful her role models, she will still need to look within herself in order to come to terms with the loss of her breast. Looking inside gives us an opportunity to connect with our core—that part of the self that exists separate and apart from the physical body. By making that connection, we are able to tap into a source of wisdom and strength which we may have been unaware of in the past. When we become aware of the core self, we can appreciate the essence of who we really are, an essence that remains safe and unscathed through all of life's vicissitudes. After my surgery, as I struggled with issues of body image, self-worth, and self-acceptance, I can remember clearly how my relationship with my own core self began to develop. Eventually, a visual image of it evolved. I saw it as a bright golden rod that seemed to be anchored deep inside my chest. I knew that my femininity was safe within that core, and no amount of physical change could ever alter it.

Many of us are unaccustomed to looking inside ourselves for answers because we are, for the most part, an outer-directed society. Hedda was a solid, down-to-earth type of woman in her mid-thirties, who lived with her lover, Ian, his two young children, and her own two-year-old son. She had joined one of my eight-week support groups after having undergone bilateral mastectomies. During the course of the group, she focused mostly on family issues, touching briefly on how she missed her breasts when she was cuddling with the children. Although she seemed to enjoy the group, for the most part she kept her feelings to herself. Two months later, I received a phone call from her. She was in considerable distress, had been feeling very angry, and was having trouble with Ian because he simply was not paying enough attention to her. She suspected that this had something to do with breast cancer, and wanted to see me. We set up an appointment for the following week.

When she arrived at my office, Hedda immediately launched into a tirade about Ian and how much more she needed from him than she had been getting. Although Ian was trying to be as considerate as possible, it seemed that Hedda's appetite for attention just could not be satisfied. As we talked, it became clear that the worse she felt about her body and her loss, the more she looked to him to take away the hurt, the sadness, and the anger. Finally, I asked her to take a moment and think about what she really wanted. Very quietly, she said, "I wish everything could be the way it was before cancer. I can't bear the fact that I must live the rest of my life without my breasts. I am not me anymore. How can I go on?"

Convinced that the answer to her question lay within herself, I asked whether she would be willing to participate in some guided imagery. Having already been exposed to some relaxation and visualization techniques in the group, Hedda readily agreed. Using a method she was already familiar with, I put her into a state of deep relaxation and then asked her to imagine herself in a safe and lovely place and report what she saw and felt.

"I am sitting on the deck of my mountain cabin," she began. "It's very beautiful up here, and very peaceful. I can see for miles. The hills are covered with redwood trees, and the air smells fresh and wonderful. The sky is a deep blue, and a gentle breeze is blowing."

"As you look around," I said, "see if there is anything in the scene that particularly draws your attention."

It was a moment before she continued. "There is a tree about fifty feet from the deck. It's an enormous redwood, and it is very special. There's a big hole right through the middle. The hole was burned into it when the tree was struck by lightning several years ago."

"Tell me your thoughts and feelings as you focus on the tree," I prompted.

"It reminds me of an old soldier who has faced many campaigns," she reflected. "With all his wounds, he continues to fight on, winning one battle after another because of his experience, his wisdom, and his patience. There is something incredibly valiant and noble about this tree. Despite the piece that's missing, it continues to grow and flourish."

Hedda had answered her own question! As she slowly opened her eyes, she said, "I guess what I really needed was to spend some time alone." Two things had become clear to her. First, her desperate longing for attention and the emptiness she had been experiencing could only be satisfied by communicating with her inner self. Any attempt to get someone else to fill that void would be futile. Second, she already had within herself much of the insight and the wisdom she needed for her own emotional healing.

Getting inside yourself is not a difficult process, but for many people it is unfamiliar. As Hedda's story illustrates, imagery is a wonderful vehicle for making contact with your own inner wisdom. There are many ways that problems of body image can be addressed through imagery. One way is simply to trust, as I did with Hedda, that whatever image comes up will be relevant to the problem. Then simply allow the image to unfold. Another approach is to invite an image of your body to appear in your mind, and then carry on a dialogue with that image. Yet a third approach is to imagine an inner adviser,* a kind, wise, and loving being who knows you very well. Your inner adviser then becomes a reliable source of comfort, reassurance, insight, and altered perspectives, and can prove helpful in many situations. Be sure not to undermine the process by having unrealistic expectations. It often takes many imagery experiences, all

---

* For specific instructions in these techniques, please refer to *Healing Yourself*, by Martin L. Rossman, M.D.

focused on different aspects of the same problem, to achieve a satisfactory resolution.

When people try to force a connection with the inner self, they usually are not successful. The process is one that requires gentleness and a willingness to sit still for your feelings. Even if you do not choose to use imagery, you can certainly make that connection by setting aside time to put yourself in a quiet place, relax, and allow your thoughts and feelings to surface. To help the process along, I often recommend that people begin with the following breathing meditation:

Find a comfortable place to sit where you will not be disturbed. Make sure your clothing is not binding you and that your arms and legs are uncrossed. Allow your eyes to close, and focus on your breathing. Each time you inhale, repeat the words "I am" to yourself. Do this for as long as it takes to establish a comfortable rhythm to your breathing. When this feels natural, add the word "okay" each time you exhale. Continue to inhale ("I am") and exhale ("okay") for a few minutes.

After several minutes of breathing meditation, you will notice that you feel considerably more relaxed. Then, let yourself gently focus on the issue that is troubling you. Without making any judgments or screening the material, just notice what comes up. Simply treat everything as valuable information that will give you better insight into yourself and your situation. As with imagery, it is unrealistic to expect a full and immediate resolution to a serious issue after only one or two attempts. It may happen that way, but usually this is a process which evolves over a period of time. Using this technique consistently helps gradually to increase your sense of well-being and self-worth. If, however, you find that your concerns about body image persist, it is important to join a breast cancer support group or to consult a professional counselor who is familiar with this particular issue.

As important as self-acceptance is, very often we need the acceptance of others to reinforce it. Theoretically, as independent adults, we should be able to maintain a positive self-image regardless of the feedback we get from others. Practically speaking, this is unrealistic. When we are subjected to either physical or emotional stress, we all tend to regress. Rather than functioning as adults, we begin to perceive and process as if we were children once again.

To understand why being accepted by others is so important, imagine a four-year-old coming home from kindergarten carrying her very first finger painting. She dashes into her house and cries excitedly, "Mommy, look what I did!" She obviously feels good about herself and is eager for her mother's reaction. What would happen if her mother answered, "That's not a very good drawing. Your cousin Sally really knows how to do a nice job." How long do you think that little girl would be able to hold on to her good feelings? If, on the other hand, that mother had said, "Yes, that's a beautiful drawing, and I'm very proud of you," the little girl would have felt entitled to keep her positive feelings. A child needs someone outside herself to reflect and reinforce her own "okayness." That gives her permission to internalize and integrate a positive self-image so that it becomes part of her inner reality.

When we deal with the loss of a breast, we must realize that our inner child is asking somewhat fearfully, "Am I okay?" While part of that answer must come from within, it is also important and valuable to get reinforcement from others about our acceptability. When you do reach out to others, be careful to choose people who are reliable, solid, kind, and compassionate. In the early stages of coming to terms with a changed body, it helps to have other people let you know that you are truly acceptable. However, ultimately, it is your own image of yourself that counts.

There is often a connection between body image, self-acceptance, and self-worth. When there is work to be done in these areas, it must take place on a deeply emotional level, almost always involving the "inner child" in some way. One of the ways to bypass the intellect and reach the "inner child" directly is through storytelling. I have been telling my patients stories for years, usually experiences of other patients who had gone through similar situations. When I studied hypnosis, I learned that myths, allegories, fables, and fairy tales can be just as effective as true stories. The unconscious mind is very aware of the task at hand, and will extract from a story exactly what is needed to speed the process of healing and growth. One day, as I was on my way to the office to see a breast cancer patient who was struggling with issues of body image and self-worth, a fairy tale wrote itself in my mind. During our session, I told her the tale, and it seemed to have a profound effect on her. Since then, sharing the story with the women in my breast cancer groups has become a tradition.

THE LITTLE GIRL AND THE SACK

Once upon a time there was a little girl who lived all alone in a small village. She was sad and lonely and desperately needed some love. One day she set out on a quest to find a way to fill the emptiness she felt inside. Before she left her home, she took a very large sack—large enough to hold as much love as she would ever need—and slung it over her shoulder. Bravely marching out into what looked like a very big world, she started down the lane, heading toward the home of her nearest neighbors. Very timidly, she rapped on the door. The door was opened by a harried-looking woman in a huge white apron. "May I help you?" she asked. "Yes, please," said the little girl. "You see, I have decided that I must have some love, so I have come out into the wide world to hunt for it. Do you have any to spare?" The woman thought for a moment and said, "I'm sorry to say that love has been in rather short supply around here lately, and we truly have none to give away. However, I happen to have this lovely old clock, and you might enjoy watching it as time passes. Will that do?" The little girl, who knew how important it was to be polite, said that she would be happy to accept the clock and thanked the woman very much. She put the clock into the big sack and continued her journey.

The next house she came to looked rather luxurious. The shutters were painted bright blue, and there was a lovely flower garden behind a white picket fence. "This is so pretty," thought the little girl. "The people who live here must be very happy. Surely they will have some love to spare."

So, once again, she knocked on a door, hoping to find enough love to make her sad and lonely feelings go away. The door was answered by a portly old gentleman with white hair and a very sad face. He listened to her request and said, "Well, my dear, I'm afraid looks are often deceiving. Our house is lovely on the outside, but the truth is that there's very little love in here, and we are all desperately trying to hold on to what little we have. There is certainly none we can afford to give away. However, I do understand your plight, and I would very much like to help you. I have an old book here—one that has been in the family for many years. I would like you to have it." Once again, the little girl said a very polite thank-you and put the book into her sack.

This time, as she walked away from the pretty house, she wondered why she was feeling even sadder and lonelier than she had before. She thought she might be hungry, so she sat down and had a bite of lunch. That didn't seem to change the way she felt at all. Telling herself that she was probably just tired from her first morning's adventures, she decided to take a nap. She found a weeping willow with branches that hung almost to the ground. She curled up in its shade and went to sleep.

Day after day she continued to search for enough love to take away her sad and lonely feelings. Day after day the results were the same—no love but more things to add to her sack. Every day the sack she was carrying grew heavier and heavier. One day she started out again and found, much to her dismay, that the sack had grown so heavy she could not lift it over her shoulder. In fact, she could not even drag it behind her on the ground. Finally, after struggling with it for a long time, she sat down, put her head in her hands, and began to weep.

After a while she lifted her tearstained face, looked down the road, and saw a stranger approaching. It was a woman with long flowing white hair just the color of moonbeams and a shimmering silver robe that shone with the light of a thousand stars. The little girl had never seen anyone like her before, but she thought the woman looked very kind and wise. The woman, whose name was Mira, sat down beside the little girl and asked why she was so sad. The little girl described her search for love, and told Mira how sad and lonely she had been. She tried to explain how important it was for her to persevere. The sack was just too heavy for her to carry any longer, and she was terrified that she would be unable to continue her quest.

Very gently, Mira asked the little girl if she could leave the sack behind. How distressed the poor child was when she heard that question! "I could never leave the sack behind," she exclaimed, "for if I do not find the love that I need, I will be left with nothing, and then I will surely die." Then Mira asked if the little girl would at least show her the things she had collected in her big sack. The little girl reached into the sack and pulled out the old clock. As soon as the sunlight touched it, the strangest thing happened. The clock turned to dust, and blew away in the breeze. Next, the little girl held up the book, and the very same thing happened. Just as soon as the sunlight touched it, the book crumbled, turned to dust, and blew away. The little girl went through the whole sack until it was completely empty. Not one of the things she had dragged around with her for all those weeks was left. Then, too scared to even cry, she looked at Mira with profound despair.

Mira smiled at her and said, "Now, my dear child, I have a gift for you. There is only one condition you must agree to before you accept it. You must promise never to put it into your sack." When the little girl nodded, Mira reached out her hand, touched the little girl's heart, and drew out from it a tiny bird. It was a most wonderful creature. Its feathers were iridescent, and when the sun touched it, the bird glistened with all the colors of the rainbow. As the little girl watched, wide-eyed, the bird hopped up onto her shoulder and began to sing the most wonderful song she had ever heard. As the bird sang, the little girl noticed that all the sad, lonely, empty feelings she had were beginning to melt away.

Mira smiled as she saw the joy of the song reflected in the little girl's face. She put her hand gently on the child's head and said, "The song you hear is your very own heartsong. It has always been there, and it will be there forever. All you have to do is listen. It will accompany you on every journey you ever decide to make in life." Then she kissed the little girl, got up to leave, and added, "There is one last thing you need to do before you continue down the road of your choice. You must decide whether you will take the empty sack with you or leave it behind." And as she walked away, the little bird's song grew clearer and ever more beautiful.

chapter ten

□

SEXUALITY

"*i*'ve made up my mind that

my husband and I will never make love again!" Anne told the group. She was fifty-five years old and had undergone a mastectomy a month before the group began. In thirty-five years of marriage, she and her husband had always had a very active and satisfying sex life, and they both took great pride in her very ample breasts. Now Anne was terrified that while they were making love her husband's hand might slip off her remaining breast and inadvertently come to rest on the flat side of her chest. She was convinced that he would be revolted by her new contour and would reject her. At a time when she was feeling very shaky about herself, it was impossible for her to believe that anyone could find her sexy, including her husband. However, it was easy to see that the prospect of giving up the intimacy that they had enjoyed over many years was terribly distressing to her.

Rather than attempting to persuade her to change her mind, I decided to use an indirect approach. I asked whether she was opposed to all sexual intimacy at this point or whether she was simply trying to protect herself. Anne stated clearly that she was afraid to let her husband touch her and couldn't bear the thought that he might see her without her nightgown on. She didn't really want to give up sex permanently but couldn't figure out how to be intimate with her husband without the risk of turning him off. Then I asked whether she had any objection to touching or pleasuring her husband. When she said she had none, I told her I might have a way out of her dilemma. Naturally, she was very much interested.

I proposed that she ask her husband to agree to a set of ground rules that would be put into effect immediately. First, she would always wear a nightgown with a bra and her prosthesis underneath to bed. Second, he was allowed to be naked whenever he wished, but he was absolutely never to suggest that she disrobe. Third, she would touch or caress him anywhere he wished, but he was not to touch her at all.

Anne liked the rules, and went home enthusiastic about establishing the new regime. After one week, she reported back to the group to say that she was pleased with the way things were going. The next week, the report was even more uplifting. The third week, she appeared in group looking very sheepish and was uncharacteristically silent. Finally, she admitted to the group that, having become very involved in their lovemaking, she had removed her nightgown herself, much to her husband's delight. When we asked whether her husband had reacted as badly as she had anticipated, she said, "Actually, it wasn't like that at all. In fact, it was really a very lovely experience—close and warm. But, best of all, when we had finished making love and were lying in bed holding each other, he whispered, "Sweetheart, I don't really miss your breast, but I missed you terribly."

In my work, I have most often encountered husbands who have been loving and supportive, but this is not always the case. Corinne, an attractive, dark-haired woman in her late fifties, attended one of my breast cancer workshops two years ago. These workshops start at nine o'clock in the morning and run until three-thirty in the afternoon with very few breaks. With twenty-five breast cancer patients all trying to share their fears and concerns in the space of a little more than six hours, the day is always packed with emotional intensity. Although Corinne said nothing for most of the day, it was clear from her body language and her facial expressions that she was very much involved in the proceedings. She paid especially close attention any time the discussion turned to body image, sexuality, or self-esteem. As the workshop drew to a close, I encouraged anyone who still had concerns that she had not yet expressed to speak up before we adjourned. It was then that Corinne finally shared her painful story.

"It has been thirteen years since my mastectomy," she began. "From the time of my surgery, my husband has never once made love to me. All this time, I believed that his reaction was perfectly reasonable. I assumed that I could no longer be considered sexual because I was now only half a woman. In all these years, it never once occurred to me that the problem might be his and not mine. I never knew about groups like this, and I never had other women to share with before." The tears that she had been choking back all day began to fall as she continued, "Today I feel as though a terrible burden has been lifted from my shoulders. For the first time in thirteen years, I feel like a person again."

When Corinne finished, I asked her to describe what her marriage had been like before she was treated for breast cancer. As I suspected, a picture of a very dysfunctional relationship began to emerge. Her husband had always been an angry man, very domineering, impatient, and perfectionistic. Corinne had often felt intimidated by his harshness and his criticisms and had spent much of her marriage trying unsuccessfully to please him. The dynamics that existed in their relationship had been well established long before Corinne's mastectomy. I suggested to Corinne that she explore the reasons she had remained in such a destructive relationship for so many years and that she try to understand her reasons for getting involved with her husband in the first place. I encouraged her to use the insight she had gained during the course of the workshop as a starting point for some serious introspection and personal growth.

When women tell me that they have fears about their sexuality and their desirability after having been treated for breast cancer, I assure them that this is a normal reaction. These feelings can be resolved fairly rapidly with some work on body image, self-worth, and communication skills. However, when women tell me about being rejected by a partner because of breast cancer, I become skeptical. If it is an established relationship, invariably there were serious problems long before breast cancer appeared. If it is a new relationship, the woman will generally admit to the fact, when pressed, that she chooses her partners unwisely. Once you feel that you deserve to have nurturing and satisfying relationships, the choices you make tend to provide you with partners who are loyal, dependable, caring, and supportive.

This past year, I ran a support group for the husbands of breast cancer patients. Jake, a transplanted New Yorker in his mid-sixties, was a kind, gentle man with a wonderful sense of humor. He was deeply concerned about his wife, who was undergoing chemotherapy at the time. She had been having a difficult time with body image, and he blamed himself. Years ago, when they were newlyweds, Florence had begun asking Jake, teasingly, why he had married her. He had always responded, "Because of your big, gorgeous, sexy breasts." This bit of banter, which had pleased them both, had been maintained lovingly through the years. Then, quite suddenly, Florence was diagnosed with breast cancer and had to have a mastectomy. Jake was torturing himself, convinced that his remark had added considerably to his wife's distress. He was afraid Florence would think he no longer desired her.

"Jake," I asked, "even on the outside chance that you married Florence only for her breasts, is that the reason you have stayed with her for all these years?"

"Of course not!" he replied indignantly.

"Will you tell me why you have stayed with her?" I went on.

"She's a wonderful woman—a great wife, a terrific mother and grandmother. She is interested in many things, and she's exciting to be with. She's my best friend. She's loyal and supportive and has never let me down. I admire her mind and I respect her values . . . and she makes a wonderful pot roast!"

I encouraged Jake to go home and share those feelings with his wife. The following week, Florence walked into the women's group looking very cheerful. "My husband said the loveliest things to me the other night," she told us, beaming. "Of course, I already knew everything he told me, but I really needed to be reminded. It made a difference."

While married women are concerned that their altered appearance will turn their husbands off, single women are terrified that they will have no place in the dating world, that they will be unable to compete, and that no man will ever want them. Sally was a tall, attractive, unattached thirty-four-year-old who had come to a breast cancer group primarily to resolve her concerns about sex and being single.

"Although I was eager to begin dating fairly soon after my mastectomy," Sally began, "I have been very worried about being rejected because I only have one breast. Even though I am coming to terms with the changes in my own body, the idea of having someone else recoil when I am at my most vulnerable is frightening. Casual dates are no problem. I have never been concerned about being good company with my clothes on. Now I'm dating someone I think I could get seriously involved with, and I find myself facing a real dilemma. What if the relationship continues to evolve? What if there is a chance of becoming physically intimate? I find myself growing more and more uncomfortable as time goes on, and I don't know what to do about it."

I explained to Sally that telling the truth was the only way out of her predicament. The group helped her define what she needed to say, and then gave her several opportunities to role-play so that she could become more comfortable with it.

The following week, a triumphant Sally walked into group. "I can't believe how well everything went!" she exclaimed. "Pete had taken me to a lovely restaurant. We had a wonderful dinner and were lingering over coffee when suddenly I knew that I had to say something. I gathered up all my courage and said, 'Pete, we've been seeing each other for a while. I like you very much, and it's possible that this relationship could develop into something really serious, so there's something I need to tell you. Several months ago, I had breast cancer and one of my breasts was removed. If you find this very disturbing, please be honest. I'm still feeling a bit fragile and self-conscious about it. I would rather end our relationship now than run the risk being rejected because of my surgery if and when we become physically intimate.' "

The group members were totally absorbed by Sally's recital, each one wondering how she would have felt in that situation. After pausing for a moment to catch her breath, Sally continued, "Pete was so wonderful! He told me that he cares for me a great deal, and that being with me makes him feel very good. As far as he's concerned, I've got more, not less, than many of the women he has dated. He said that who I am is far more meaningful to him than how many breasts I have, and he's looking forward to us getting closer in many ways, including physically."

In general, I find that men come through beautifully, if we let them. Unfortunately, when women send out signals about how terrible they feel, and how they don't want to be seen, much less touched, men may back off for fear of hurting or embarrassing their partners. Women can misinterpret that as a message about how unacceptable they are. Even after several months, some women still hide from their partners. There are two issues here. First, it is unrealistic to expect a man to have no reaction whatsoever to the fact that his wife or lover has lost a breast. Breasts are a lovely part of an intimate relationship, bringing pleasure to both partners. It is quite appropriate for a man to feel a real sense of loss should his partner lose one or both of her breasts. However, a truly intimate relationship hinges on far more than a woman's breasts. Most of the men I have spoken to tell me that any loss they may feel is temporary, and they are much more concerned with their partner's life than with her breast(s). Second, if it is hard for a woman to confront her altered appearance for the first time, her partner deserves some latitude as well. It's not fair to expect a man to adjust to a significant change in his partner's body and feel sexual all at the same time. When a woman is having difficulty showing her partner her surgery, I will recommend that they find a place away from the bedroom where they can help each other discuss, look, and touch in a completely nonsexual way. That way, they can become reacquainted as they both adapt to the changes in her body. It is very important not to make sex a goal at this time, but to reach out to each other in comforting, reassuring ways that are indicative of a different kind of intimacy.

Many women will ask to see photographs of mastectomies before they have their own surgery. The trouble is that most pictures in medical texts and journals are singularly unattractive. They are taken just after surgery, when the scars are quite red and pronounced, and the surrounding area is discolored or swollen. In addition, the women in the photographs are either shown from the neck down, or their eyes, nose, and mouth are blacked out to protect their identity. For the most part, they seem to convey feelings of sadness, vulnerability, and embarrassment. However, there is a wonderful poster available which most doctors are unaware of. It is a photograph of Deena Metzger, a feminist poet and author, standing nude in the bright sunlight, arms outflung, head thrown back, radiating joy and sensuality. The only thing unusual about this photograph is that it was taken after Deena had her mastectomy. If you want a positive image of what it looks like to be one-breasted, I recommend this poster without reservation.* I often suggest that women with mastectomies who feel awkward about being seen by their partner show the poster first. That way, they can both become accustomed to the look of a one-breasted woman without either of them feeling too exposed or too vulnerable.

If you find yourself feeling shaky about your sexuality, you might also go back and reread the chapter on Body Image. Many times, the problem really lies in the area of self-image rather than sexuality. I recently ran a group for couples where the wives were being treated for breast cancer. The husbands unanimously agreed that their reaction to their wives' altered appearance was minimal. Their overriding concerns had to do with fear of losing their mates as a result of the disease, their own feelings of helplessness and confusion in the face of their wives' emotional turmoil, and treatment side effects. Of course, they were aware of how distressed and upset their spouses were about their loss of a breast(s). The husbands simply did not share those feelings. Several of the men had tried to reassure their wives about this, and were not believed. No matter how open and accepting your partner is, if you are convinced that no one could ever find you attractive or sexual without one or both of your breasts,

---

* Posters and brochures can be ordered from TREE, P.O. Box 186, Topanga, CA 90290.

then you will continue to have a problem. I do encourage women who find it difficult to resolve this issue on their own to find a counselor or therapist. A caring and competent professional can provide the support necessary to help you move past a place where you may feel stuck.

As always, meeting with women who have moved past this stage in their recovery and feel good about themselves and their sexuality is extremely valuable at this time. It helps to know that recovery is possible. Use the resource list in Appendix B to make some of those connections. Also, it is important to understand that the more you hide and the more you indulge your reluctance to face this issue in a straightforward way, the more convinced you will become that you must step out of the sexual arena. Whether you have a brand-new partner or one with whom you have had a longstanding relationship, the issue can be dealt with, discussed and resolved together.

A few months after my mastectomy, I attended a breast cancer support group led by a social worker named Jean. She was a recovered breast cancer patient who had undergone surgery over twenty years before. Her mastectomy was performed at a time when the surgery was far more extensive than the modified radical mastectomy that is considered standard treatment today. During the fifth session, she announced that it had always been her practice to invite her participants to show each other their surgery. Without exception, the twelve women in the group turned white, all of us feeling shocked, nervous, and quite threatened. Jean explained that many women had never seen a mastectomy on anyone else. Their first encounter with such an altered appearance was their own surgery. Because there was no basis for comparison, many women were left feeling painfully different, isolated, and unacceptable. In her experience, when women had a chance to look at each other, they felt much less lonely and much less different. Their self-confidence would begin to build the moment they saw that they were not alone. Jean pointed out that she was not trying to be cruel or sadistic. The only reason she had continued the practice was because the results were so beneficial. To give everyone time to adjust and to decide whether to participate, Jean went first.

Once she had removed her blouse and her bra, Jean began to tell us what she liked about her body. Her mastectomy had been on the left side, and she pointed to a spot between two ribs where we could see a delicate pulsing. It was her heart! From the first moment Jean became aware that she could see the beating of her heart, she had been entranced. She had felt a combination of awe, gratitude, and and a deep appreciation of both her fragility and her strength. She went on describing her body in very loving terms, and then said something that had a lasting impact on me. "When I make love," she told us, "one of the most intimate things my lover can do is to caress the side of my chest where I have had the surgery. The love, the acceptance, and the tenderness that are conveyed in that gesture make me feel incredibly close to him, and I find that very sexy." I found her experience touching and valuable, and I have passed it on to all the women who have participated in my groups since then. Just as a point of information, when Jean was through, we all did remove our shirts. As it turned out, she was absolutely right. Many of us went home that night feeling so high that we couldn't get to sleep until the wee hours of the morning!

There are some women who are accustomed to achieving sexual arousal primarily through breast and nipple stimulation. When they must undergo bilateral mastectomies (removal of both breasts), they sometimes feel sexually disoriented and deprived. For these women and their partners, I recommend the Masters and Johnson technique called "sensate focus." Sensate focus is really a program of mutual exploration, the one condition being that genitals and breasts are off-limits. The advantage of this technique is that it allows a woman to focus on other areas of her body that can afford her great sensual pleasure and actually allow her to reprogram her sexual responses. If a couple finds it difficult or awkward to use this program, a few sessions with a qualified sex therapist can prove invaluable.

Women who are being treated for breast cancer will sometimes report a drastic reduction in sexual interest, which may have nothing to do with an alteration in appearance. An active involvement in lovemaking takes some energy, and both chemotherapy and radiation can cause considerable fatigue. In addition, chemotherapy may play havoc with the biochemistry of the entire body, including the hormonal balance. Depression, whether it is chemically induced or just a normal response to breast cancer diagnosis and treatment, can also cause a marked loss of libido (sex drive). Women tend to find this upsetting and often fear that an essential part of their vitality has been lost forever. It is reassuring for them to learn that this loss of interest in sex is temporary. Once treatment is completed, physical and emotional recovery should progress fairly rapidly, and women can expect to return to their normal level of sexual functioning.

Women also express concern about how their lack of interest in sex will affect their partners. It can be very confusing for a man to reach out to his partner sexually, not only to reassure her that she is still attractive and desirable, but also to maintain a sense of closeness and connection during a time that seems very threatening, only to have her pull away. He may feel hurt, rejected, angry, and helpless. He, too, must be reassured that the situation is temporary and is not a reflection of his partner's feelings toward him. It is also important for both partners to appreciate that there are ways to connect physically that are nonsexual. Women often tell me that their most pressing need is to be held and hugged, but are concerned that their partners will be offended if this is not an invitation to lovemaking. I always encourage these women to communicate their needs directly to their partners. Not only are the men relieved to find that they are not being rejected, but they also feel pleased and proud that there is something of value they can offer their partner that will help her to feel more secure, loved, and protected.

chapter eleven

RECONSTRUCTION

i was forty-one-years-old and single when my surgeon informed me that I would need a mastectomy. The doctor was as gentle as possible, but I remember feeling overwhelming terror and despair. How could I live the rest of my life without one of my breasts? I was afraid I would never be able to adapt to the change in my own body—afraid I would never really like myself again. In the unlikely event that I did somehow come to terms with the loss, I was convinced that no one else would ever find me acceptable. I didn't know very much about breast reconstruction at the time, but it seemed the one hope I had of preserving myself as a woman. When I asked my surgeon about it, he told me that immediate reconstruction was out of the question because of the radiation therapy I had undergone three-and-a-half years before. He was concerned that the radiation might have damaged the circulation in the chest area and might cause some difficulties in healing after my surgery. His recommendation was that I delay any reconstruction at least six months, giving my skin and muscle ample opportunity to heal. I trusted his judgment implicitly, and agreed to wait the six months, but I was absolutely determined to have the procedure the moment he gave his approval.

Until I was discharged from the hospital, I avoided looking at myself. The day I came home, I stood in front of my bathroom mirror, determined to have a look. I chided myself for feeling so cowardly as I slowly unbuttoned my pajama top and exposed my chest. Although I had known for weeks that I would be left without a breast, I had managed to resist the temptation to conjure up any pictures in my mind. Losing my breast had been an abstraction until this moment. Now, staring at my reflection in the mirror, I was devastated by the radical change in my own body. I felt a tremendous wave of nausea, and then the room started to spin. I didn't know whether I was going to throw up or pass out. In the end, I did neither. Instead, I lay down on the floor, curled up into a little ball, and wept.

I knew I would be able to have reconstruction after six months, but in those early days following my mastectomy, the time seemed to stretch endlessly into the future. In the meantime, I was anxious to go on with my life. As I began to heal both physically and emotionally, I noticed something rather surprising. Each day, I found myself feeling just a little better about my body. Somehow, the fact that I had survived a recurrence of cancer as well as a very threatening surgery added to my self-confidence. Within a fairly short time, I began dating. I discovered that I was relating to men in a different and better way. I found myself much more attracted to men who had special qualities such as warmth, sensitivity, and openness. I felt shy and scared the first time I became intimately involved with a man, but we had already become very good friends and my missing breast did not distress him in the least. That was quite a revelation to me. I had grown up believing that my facade had to be perfect for me to be acceptable. What I discovered was that there was a real me that could be seen, appreciated, and valued by others and was definitely unaffected by how many breasts I had. I began to realize that my femininity and my sexuality were intact, even though my body was not, and that my changed appearance didn't bar me from experiencing closeness and intimacy.

As the months went by, I thought less and less about reconstruction. Then one day I was in my surgeon's office for a routine checkup. He remarked that my wound had healed very well, and asked me if

I was ready for reconstruction. Recalling how desperately I had wanted it at the time of my mastectomy, he expected me to be elated. With a shock, I realized that almost a year had passed. Much to our mutual surprise, I told him that I would like to think about it for a while. When I went home that afternoon, I spent hours arguing with myself about the pros and cons of restorative surgery. Finally, I realized that it simply wasn't necessary for me. I was feeling good about myself, I had proof that I was acceptable to others, and I was content. I had come to terms with my loss, and my body image was a positive one. Because my missing breast was not causing me any real emotional distress, I did not feel motivated to undergo any further surgery.

My decision not to have breast reconstruction was not a matter of settling for second best. I did a great deal of work on myself in the year following my mastectomy, and I paid careful attention to the issues pertaining to body image. First, I refused to hide from myself. I learned to look at myself in the mirror, confronting my altered appearance regularly until my uneasiness began to subside. Once I felt a little steadier, I arranged to have the most important women in my life look at my surgery. I desperately needed to hear that they still found me acceptable. Once that was accomplished, I was able to venture out a little further. While on vacation, I arranged to have a massage and nervously told the masseuse about my mastectomy. I expected her to cancel our appointment, thinking that she would be too scared or repulsed to deal with me. Much to my surprise, she said, "Dearie, I've been in this business a long time and I've seen it all. Nothing bothers me!" I found that very comforting.

I challenged myself to redefine sexuality, femininity, and beauty. It took time to separate myself from society's definitions of these terms, but, as I wrestled with them, I came to a very important realization. It is not the eye of the beholder that counts! I am sexy if I feel sexy. I am feminine if I feel feminine. I discovered that those feelings had to do with my own sense of myself rather than the reactions that people might have to me. Even so, the idea of having an intimate relationship with a man was still very frightening. Clearly, there was a decision to be made. I chose to risk a possible rejection rather than allow cancer to deprive me of anything in life that could bring me warmth, closeness, pleasure, and joy. The consequences of that decision have been remarkable. Since my mastectomy, the men in my life have been supportive, loving, and totally accepting. They have helped me to appreciate myself as a whole person instead of defining myself in terms of a missing breast.

Of course, in addition to the focus on my body, I was also dealing with all the other issues women confront during and after a breast cancer experience: mortality, fear of recurrence, powerlessness, communication problems, and a bewildering range of emotions. By the time a year had passed, I had done so much work on myself and had undergone such profound changes that a fascinating thing began to happen. I would stand in front of the mirror, look at my chest, and feel an enormous sense of pride. Somehow, the scar from my mastectomy had become my badge—a reminder of the many victories I had won as I had confronted and resolved one issue after another. At that point, not only did the idea of reconstruction become unnecessary for me but I found that I had grown very much attached to my new look. I was not willing to give up my badge.

I am often asked how I can enthusiastically support a woman's decision to have breast reconstruction when I have adjusted so well to being one-breasted. First of all, I applaud any decision that moves a woman in the direction of emotional healing, increased self-confidence, and a sense of joy and freedom. Most of my patients who have opted for reconstruction are delighted with the results and agree that the surgery has had a very positive impact on their lives. In view of the marvelous success stories that I have heard, it would be both presumptuous and arrogant of me to insist that my way is the only way. Second, like so many of the women I have treated, I was terrified at the prospect of losing my breast. At the time of my mastectomy, the only thing that I found in any way comforting was my doctor's assurance that I could have reconstruction some time in the future. As it turned out, I came to terms with my body in a way I could never have predicted at the time. However, the lessons I learned about self-worth and acceptability are applicable to all my breast cancer patients, whether or not they have had reconstruction.

While I ultimately chose not to have restorative surgery, knowing that it was an option helped me through some very dark and painful times.

Whether or not a woman opts for reconstruction, which type(s) of surgery she may choose, and the timing of that surgery are complex issues involving both medical and emotional considerations. (For a brief explanation of the medical and technical aspects of breast reconstruction, please refer to Appendix F.) Women who decide in favor of reconstruction may do so for a variety of reasons. Wendy was an articulate, assertive twenty-eight-year-old who was already rising in the ranks of a major corporation. Her looks were as dramatic as her personality, and she had a beautiful figure. She had been diagnosed with breast cancer a few months before she came to one of my groups, and had been treated with a mastectomy and immediate reconstruction. Many of the women in the group were curious about the surgery, and Wendy was most willing to share her experiences.

"When my surgeon told me that I would need a mastectomy, he asked whether I would like to consider immediate reconstructive surgery. The minute he suggested it, I knew it was for me. I'm young, single, and I have my whole life ahead of me. If I can, I want to live it with my body intact, or at least with some sense of physical wholeness. It was hard enough to deal with the idea that I have cancer, and worse to think that I would be forced to lose one of my breasts. I was terrified of going back into the dating scene feeling awkward and self-conscious. It's very competitive out there, and I felt that I would be at a distinct disadvantage if I were missing a breast. If I could wake up from surgery already "under construction," I knew it would make the loss easier to bear. I am thrilled with my new breast. At first I was afraid that it would feel alien, but it has really become an integral part of my body. I know that the decision I made is not for everyone, but I am absolutely delighted, and for me it was the right way to go."

The advantage of immediate reconstruction is that it avoids the most severe psychological trauma associated with the loss of a breast. However, it is by no means mandatory that restorative surgery be performed at the time of a mastectomy. It can be performed any-where from a few days to many years later. There are many women who had mastectomies at a time when breast reconstruction was not available, and they, too, are candidates for restorative surgery. **You are never too old, and it is never too late!** If restoration of the body's integrity is meaningful to a twenty-eight-year-old woman, there is no reason why it should not be just as meaningful to a sixty-eight-year-old. It saddens me when I hear people referring to breast reconstruction as a surgery that is motivated by vanity. Once our breasts develop, it is perfectly natural to expect to keep them for the rest of our lives. The yearning of a breast cancer patient to return in some way to physical wholeness is very understandable, and de-serves to be treated with compassion. If a woman chooses breast restoration, it must be considered an important part of her physical and emotional recovery.

The arguments in favor of immediate reconstruction are certainly compelling. However, there are many situations where a delayed procedure is the surgery of choice. Some doctors recommend a post-ponement of a few months in order to obtain a better cosmetic result. Sometimes a woman is not a candidate for a simple implant procedure (see Appendix E) and must be somewhat recovered from her mas-tectomy before one of the more complex flap procedures can be used. In addition, if the woman needs further treatment, such as chemotherapy, her physicians may advise that reconstruction not be done until her treatment is completed. Aside from the medical con-siderations, many women feel that they are much too overwhelmed at the time of diagnosis to do full justice to the issue of reconstruction. They prefer to get the preliminary surgery out of the way, and then focus their attention on educating themselves and interviewing plastic surgeons. They want to have the opportunity to make decisions about reconstruction at a time when they are not under the pressure of a cancer diagnosis or treatment, and can feel much calmer, more secure, and much more in command of the situation.

My friend Abby is a Reach to Recovery volunteer. I met her when I first started leading breast cancer groups for the American Cancer Society. Abby is a transplanted New Yorker in her early sixties, very outspoken and very assertive. Thirteen years ago, she was diagnosed with breast cancer. Abby has always been a reader and a researcher. At the time she was diagnosed, the lumpectomy was first being considered as an alternative to mastectomy. Very anxious not to lose her breast, Abby presented the possibility of a lumpectomy to her doctors, only to discover that no one was willing to perform it. She even flew from Los Angeles back to New York, hoping to find a doctor who was familiar with the new technique and confident of the outcome, but to no avail. Unfortunately, Abby was about a year too early. Although the medical community was on the verge of accepting the lumpectomy as a legitimate and effective treatment for breast cancer, the procedure was still too new to have collected a large following.

After a great deal of running around, Abby finally had her mastectomy. Her husband was very loving and supportive and never made her feel any less desirable than she had always been. However, Abby was miserable. Every time she looked at herself, she was reminded that she had had cancer. It made her feel sad, vulnerable, and often fearful. She hated feeling lopsided, and she was angry about having to wear a prosthesis in her bra. Abby was a superb athlete who swam and played tennis regularly. She found her prosthesis uncomfortable, inconvenient, and cumbersome. She was always worried that it would fall out and embarrass her while she was engaged in one of her activities. She was also a talented clothing designer, and had created a lovely wardrobe for herself. Her favorite dresses were either low-cut or strapless, and she was upset that she couldn't wear them anymore.

About three years after her mastectomy, Abby began hearing a great deal about breast reconstruction. The more she researched, the more she was convinced that this was for her. She interviewed several plastic surgeons and finally settled on the one who seemed to have the most experience with breast implants. Although she ran into a few complications and had to have the implant replaced about two years later, Abby has been delighted with the results of her surgery. She donated her prosthesis to the American Cancer Society, and marked the occasion with a cocktail party. There are no more restrictions on the kinds of clothes she wears, and she feels really free whenever she engages in sports. Best of all, her body no longer reminds her of cancer. While the awareness of her own vulnerability will never disappear completely, it has definitely faded into the background.

Abby was very much aware of the importance of selecting the right plastic surgeon. While some women require only that a surgeon have a reputation for technical excellence, others will not feel comfortable unless they can also establish a personal rapport with their physician. I strongly recommend that any woman seriously considering breast reconstruction interview at least two specialists before making a decision. Because there are many questions to be answered and so much information to absorb, a writing pad and/or a tape recorder can prove invaluable. It is extremely helpful to formulate a set of questions in advance. The following series of questions, though not complete, may serve as a guide:

- Which reconstructive technique(s) am I a candidate for, and why?
- Will you explain the procedure(s) along with any risks or complications?
- How many surgeries will be required? Please explain each one in detail.
- Will my remaining breast need to be operated on as well?
- Which procedures will be done in your office, and which will require hospital admission?
- How long will recuperation take at each stage, and what will my physical limitations be?
- Will the reconstruction interfere in any way with future cancer detection?
- How many surgeries of this type have you performed to date?
- Do you have any pictures to show me of the results you have obtained with other women like myself?
- Can you introduce me to one of your patients who has already completed the reconstructive process?

• How much do you charge for each of these procedures? How much of the expense is covered by health insurance?

During this investigative period, it is very important to meet and speak with women who have already undergone breast reconstruction. They can be wonderful resources, and can supply much reassurance, encouragement, and support. They will tell you about their experiences and, in most cases, also show you the results of their surgery. If your plastic surgeon cannot make such contacts available to you, your local branch of the American Cancer Society will be able to put you in touch with a Reach to Recovery volunteer who has had reconstruction.

There is one point I always stress whenever the subject of reconstruction comes up. It is simply not true that a woman must undergo restorative surgery in order to be acceptable to others. When a woman feels that way, she does a tremendous disservice to herself by seriously discounting her own worth. Sue was a petite, attractive, forty-six-year-old woman who attended one session of a breast cancer group and then phoned for a private appointment. She told me that her problems were different from those she had heard in the group, and she felt self-conscious about airing her troubles publicly. When she first arrived at my office, I was struck by her attempts to remain cheerful and businesslike. In a very matter-of-fact voice, she began filling me in on her medical history. Three years before, she had found a lump in her breast that had turned out to be malignant. At the time, she had undergone a lumpectomy and radiation and had assumed that she was cured. Two years later, she found another lump in the same breast. This time, a mammogram revealed that she had cancer in the other breast as well. Her doctors felt that it was in her best interest to undergo a double mastectomy, and Sue had agreed. It had been a year since her surgery, and she admitted that she was still having difficulties with body image.

So far I hadn't heard anything particularly unusual and began to wonder why Sue considered herself so different from other breast cancer patients. I asked her whether she had some special concerns that she hadn't yet mentioned. She was silent for a few moments, and in that short time I saw her expression change from detachment to anguish. Finally, her voice choked with pain, she sobbed, "Breast cancer is wrecking my marriage. My husband can't stand me anymore, and I don't blame him. I can't even look at myself without feeling revolted. He says I'm always depressed, and all I ever think about is cancer. I'm losing my husband, and it's all my fault! I wanted to have reconstruction. I have seen three plastic surgeons, and no one will operate on me because I've had radiation. Now my husband will probably divorce me, and there's nothing I can do about it."

Over a period of months, Sue and I addressed these issues one at a time. First we worked on body image. Once she was feeling better about her appearance, we tackled her fears about mortality, cancer, and the possibility of further recurrences. After that, we began to take a close look at her marriage. It was difficult for Sue to admit that there had been serious problems in her relationship with her husband beginning years before she had ever had breast cancer. She herself was a product of a broken home, and she had considered it vitally important that her own family remain intact. She had tried to ignore the many problems that had surfaced over the years, afraid that her security would be threatened if she ever acknowledged them. Gradually, Sue was able to resolve her childhood fears about abandonment and set aside her old feelings about the stigma that she had always believed was attached to divorce. At that point, she and her husband separated.

Within a fairly short period of time, Sue began to date. Much to her amazement, she found that she was extremely popular and her social life was very active. Eventually, she found a wonderful man who became very important to her. At that point, we began to deal with her fears about physical intimacy and rejection.

One day, Sue bounced into my office and proudly announced, "We did it!"

"It?" I asked, caught off-guard and feeling a bit confused.

"You know," she said emphatically, "IT!"

"Ah," I said, finally understanding. "And how was it?"

"Incredible," she replied. "It's the best sex I ever had. Chuck was a wonderful lover, and he wasn't turned off at all by my missing breasts. He made me feel feminine, sexy, and desirable, and I can't wait to do it again!"

When Sue had first come to see me, she had felt desolate because none of the plastic surgeons she had interviewed were willing to risk doing a breast implant. At the time, I had suggested that she do some research on a fairly new procedure called the TRAM flap (see Appendix F). In this type of reconstructive surgery, tissue is removed from the lower abdomen in an operation similar to a tummy tuck. The tissue is then transferred to the chest wall, after which it is shaped into breasts. Sue had done her homework and had found a plastic surgeon in Atlanta who was one of the nation's foremost experts in this type of procedure. A few months after she had become involved with Chuck, Sue decided to fly to Atlanta for reconstruction. "I know Chuck loves me," she explained, "and he says that I should save myself the ordeal because it isn't necessary. I appreciate that, and I'm grateful that he feels that way, but lately I keep thinking about how lovely it would be to have breasts again. I know I could get along without the surgery, and I could probably live quite happily. It's just that I have been through so much in the last few years, and I have made so many changes that I feel as though I'm starting a new life. I really want to give myself a present to mark this new beginning, and the best present I can think of is new breasts."

Sue did go on to have the surgery, which was a complete success. She is proud of herself for pursuing her goal, and absolutely delighted with the results. It was clear to her that her acceptability as a person, a woman, and a sexual partner did not hinge on how many breasts she had. However, before her reconstruction, she had always been aware of a tinge of self-consciousness during lovemaking. Eager to be rid of the last vestiges of negative feelings about her body, she had simply decided that restorative surgery was a gift she could give herself, and she knew she was worth it.

chapter twelve

THE EMOTIONAL ROLLER COASTER

*t*wo years ago, I ran a workshop for the daughters of women with breast cancer. It was there that I met Cathy, a warm and friendly woman who was trying to overcome some of the fears that had remained with her as a result of her mother's illness. Neither of us suspected then that she would be diagnosed with breast cancer less than a year later. She kept in close contact with me after her diagnosis, and it was a month after her lumpectomy that this phone conversation took place.

"I feel as though I'm on an emotional roller coaster," sobbed Cathy. "My cancer was caught very early, I didn't have to lose my breast, I recovered pretty quickly from surgery, and I can even move my arm without much trouble. I just started my radiation treatments yesterday, and they seem to be going well. I know I should feel very grateful, but something is terribly wrong. I can't get anything accomplished. The smallest task seems totally overwhelming. I haven't been able to stop crying for the last two days. I find myself bursting into tears for absolutely no reason. What's the matter with me?"

"Cathy," I said reassuringly, "there is a very good reason for your tears, and it sounds as though you are right on schedule."

"I am?" she asked, obviously quite surprised.

"It's not unusual for women to hold in their tears while they get through the most difficult part of treatment, and then really let go when things ease up a bit," I explained. "You're certainly not the first woman I've spoken to who has had to deal with some uncontrollable crying."

"That makes me feel a little more normal," she replied, "but I still don't understand what the tears are about. All the doctors were very encouraging. They tell me that my chances for a cure are better than 95 percent. Shouldn't I be feeling grateful about that?"

"You probably are," I said, "but that doesn't automatically erase all the fear, vulnerability, sadness, anger, and anxiety that you also must have been feeling over the last several weeks. Even though you're not in great danger of dying from cancer, you are still coming face to face with your own mortality. On top of that, you're probably in touch with a young inner child who is feeling kicked around, terrified, and very much overwhelmed by a world that is very unsafe. Now that things have slowed down, you finally have an opportunity to get at these feelings, and they seem to be hitting you all at once. No wonder you're crying."

As we talked, it seemed that Cathy needed to be reassured on several counts. She needed to know that her feelings were normal, that they made sense, and that the crying would not last forever. She had been measuring herself against some picture of what one *should* be feeling, and she had no idea that the picture was unrealistic.

Women who are recovering from breast cancer often feel puzzled and dismayed by what they are feeling. If their feelings do not "make sense," they begin to panic, and assume that something is wrong with them. They may feel completely out of control and perceive themselves as helpless victims of their emotions. They may be confused and bewildered by the unexpected feelings that arise. They may experience shame or guilt as they suddenly become aware of emotions society has labeled nasty, sinful, petty, sick, or vengeful. Worst of all, they sometimes fear that they are suffering from some sort of mental disorder.

I approach feelings with a great deal of respect and take the position that they *always* make sense. There is invariably a good reason for what we feel, even if the reason is not immediately apparent. Unfortunately, instead of looking inside ourselves for valuable insights, we tend to dismiss our feelings because they are not logical, or else we judge them unfairly by using "shoulds" and "oughts." It is a mistake to appoint the rational mind to be the arbiter of our emotions. The rational mind is like a computer. It is a fine instrument, designed to deal with facts in a logical way, and we depend on its problem-solving abilities. Feelings, however, are not problems to be solved, although many people attempt to treat them that way. Once they are heard, understood, accepted, and treated with compassion, feelings tend to solve themselves! Feelings are communications from the "inner child," and they have a logic of their own. We frequently experience emotions that seem to be in conflict with each other. While it may be difficult to accept or understand, these inconsistencies are an integral part of the way human beings function on an emotional level. Feelings may appear to be inconsistent, but they are never wrong.

It is also a mistake to expect your emotions to be governed by "shoulds" that have been imposed either by yourself or by those around you. We are inundated with "shoulds" from the time we are very young. They are inherited from parents and teachers, religion, society, and even from our peers. We grow up learning to distort or disguise our own emotional truths in order to accommodate ourselves to these "shoulds." Even when we are not placing restrictions on our own feelings, we are often surrounded by other people who will. I find myself frequently explaining to women in my breast cancer groups that people who try to impose rules and restrictions on what others feel may do so for any number of reasons: they may be unfamiliar with their own emotional terrain and therefore unacquainted with feelings in general; they may be unaware of the specific feelings that routinely accompany recovery from breast cancer; they may be trying to help in the only way they know; they may be afraid of a particular feeling; they may be feeling frustrated by their own helplessness. Regardless of where the "shoulds" have come from, it is important to recognize that feelings don't obey rules. Feelings simply are.

Incessant crying is just one of the many responses that women find difficult or confusing as they move through recovery from breast cancer. What follows are some of the statements made by group members, along with my own comments and explanations.

Eve, age 28, secretary

After surgery, I was really high. For weeks, I felt happy and optimistic. Everyone was amazed that I had gotten through it so well, and I was very proud of myself. My good mood lasted for two months. Then, suddenly, I woke up one morning feeling terribly depressed. I seem to have crashed, and I just can't get myself back up again. I don't understand what happened. Now that I think about it, it doesn't even make sense that I was feeling so good at the beginning.

Surgery is usually perceived as a major threat. Surviving it can often generate a feeling of euphoria that may last anywhere from a few moments to several months. In addition, many women truly enjoy the experience of being the center of attention in those first few weeks. Friends and family may express their love and concern in ways that make the recovering patient feel special—something that may be conspicuously absent in her everyday life. However, as the attention wanes, the euphoria begins to fade. Eventually, those people who have rallied in the face of the immediate crisis tend to resume their own lives and routines, confident that the patient's high spirits will last. When the excitement dies down and the distractions are gone, a woman may find herself alone with her thoughts for the first time since her surgery. Ironically, that may be just the time when she finds herself becoming aware of the very normal fears and concerns that accompany cancer diagnosis and treatment. Actually, the time alone can be a blessing in disguise. It gives a woman the opportunity to pay careful attention to her own feelings, identify those issues that are of most concern, and begin to face them. At that point, sharing with others can be especially valuable. Although time alone may be necessary in order to get in touch with your own feelings, it is very important to remember that you need not work your way through these issues alone.

Sheila, age 42, attorney

Chemotherapy was difficult for me. Sometimes I felt as though it would just go on forever. I used to count the days until treatment would be over. When I knew that I was two weeks away from my last treatment, I even began to plan a party. Well, I had my final injection three days ago, and I don't feel like celebrating at all. All I feel is sad and depressed.

Sheila's reaction is fairly common. No matter how difficult treatment may be, there is always a sense that a woman and her doctors are actively engaged in a battle against cancer. Once treatment is over, a woman may feel alone, abandoned, and totally unprotected. The reassuring connection she had with her doctor may seem threatened when she is told that weekly or monthly office visits will no longer be necessary. Without radiation or cancer-fighting chemicals, she wonders what will keep cancer at bay, and feelings of vulnerability, fear, and sadness may now emerge. These feelings are certainly understandable, and eventually they will fade. In the meantime, support from other women who are familiar with this transitional stage is especially helpful.

Beth, age 37, housewife

Last Saturday night was probably the worst time I've had since my mastectomy. Until then, I had been doing pretty well. I was able to look at myself in the mirror without becoming upset. Once I got my prosthesis, I stopped feeling self-conscious in clothes. My husband and I have resumed our lovemaking, and that has gone very well. I was confident that I was really on the road to recovery. Then I had to go to this ridiculous party. I was feeling good about myself until a woman walked in wearing a low-cut dress. I couldn't take my eyes off her cleavage. All of a sudden, I felt ugly, different, and deformed. In my mind, I heard myself wishing that she would get breast cancer too. I feel so ashamed. Knowing how terrible an experience it has been, how could I possibly wish it on anyone else? I never thought I was such an awful person!

Beth wasn't awful—just human. Human beings aren't limited to feeling love, generosity, altruism, and kindness. We also experience envy, jealousy, resentment, hostility, and many other emotions that are considered negative. The fact that we have these thoughts and feelings does not make us bad or wrong, as long as we don't act them out in ways that are hurtful to ourselves or others. Clearly, the situation was an intensely painful one. Envy is difficult to bear under any circumstances, but in this particular case, Beth was suddenly confronted with the enormity of the loss she had sustained. Believing she was on the mend, she was unprepared for the magnitude of her reaction. As we began to work this through, she came to understand that by directing her hostility at the woman with the cleavage, she was saving herself from an underlying feeling of profound grief. Once she allowed herself to truly grieve, her feelings of hostility and envy began to dissipate.

Juli, age 34, sales representative

This past week I went back to work, and five or six of my co-workers told me how fabulous I look. Before I had cancer, that would have made me feel great. When I hear it now, I just get furious. I don't understand why I should be so upset.

Juli had undergone a mastectomy two months before. She was on chemotherapy, had lost all her hair, and was feeling physically ill and exhausted. Her entire family lived two thousand miles away. She was single and terribly lonely. Juli had many fears about her prospects for marriage, the effectiveness of her treatment, and whether she would have time to accomplish some of her goals in life. When people told her that she was looking wonderful, she felt her emotional distress was being overlooked or discounted. She felt that people didn't really care and that they had no tolerance for her emotional pain. She experienced their comments on her appearance as a demand that she play a game of pretend to make them feel more comfortable. The truth is that with her wig in place and her makeup on, she did look lovely. Nevertheless, she had a very strong need for people to ask about her psychological state rather than compliment her on her physical appearance. Once she understood her own needs, she was able to choose a few co-workers and communicate truthfully to them. Happily, they responded well, and were able to be supportive throughout the rest of her treatment.

Roxanne, age 54, real estate broker

I have always been known for my wonderful sense of humor. People used to enjoy being around me because they could always count on a good laugh, no matter how serious the situation. I was always pretty even-tempered and extremely patient with people, too. Now everyone annoys me. I find myself flying off the handle at the least little thing. It's getting really hard for me to find humor in anything. I'm afraid I am turning into a real witch.

Many women are surprised and upset at the amount of anger they feel as they go through recovery from breast cancer. In Roxanne's case, we discovered a long list of reasons for this anger. She was furious that cancer had disrupted her life and forced her to put her plans on hold. She found it intolerable that her life, which had once been filled with laughter and joy, was now crowded with visits to doctors, medical terminology, uncertainty, and fear. She felt outraged that chemotherapy, which was supposed to cure her, was making her feel so sick. She was incensed that cancer had the power to turn her from the loving, giving person she had always known herself to be into an angry shrew. Most of all, she was angry at her own sense of helplessness in the face of this disease. As we began to explore together, Roxanne came to understand that she wasn't really angry with other people at all, but rather with God or fate and the unfairness of it all. At that point she was willing to acknowledge some of her other feelings, such as sadness, fear, vulnerability, and grief, and allowed herself to express them fully. As she did so, some of the anger began to abate.

An inner conflict she had been unaware of was also brought to her attention. In the past, she had been accustomed to giving a great deal of her time and attention to others. Now, she was totally absorbed in issues that affected her own survival. Without realizing it, she had started to resent the attention demanded by others, yet was unwilling to spoil her image of herself as a giving person. Once this issue was clarified, she was able to make peace with the fact that her own needs must be given priority because of the crisis at hand. She understood that this was temporary, and once treatment was over, she would be free to decide how to strike a better balance between the recognition of her own needs and her pleasure in helping others.

The list of feelings goes on and on, ranging from anger to grief, and from euphoria to immobilizing depression. Sometimes women wonder whether they will ever be able to escape from the feelings that seem to engulf them. Regardless of what the complex of emotions may be, the approach is basically the same. If you find yourself overwhelmed with a particular feeling, you can look inside yourself to gain more understanding of your inner process, look to people outside yourself for validation and support, or use a combination of both strategies. No matter which way you choose to go, start by assuring yourself that there are very good reasons for your feelings, even if those reasons are not obvious to you at the moment.

Looking inside can give you insight into your feelings, but you must be willing to sit still and allow thoughts, images, and other messages from your "inner child" to surface. The meditation and imagery techniques described in Chapter 3 (. . . And Do You Have a Teddy Bear?) and Chapter 9 (Body Image), including ways of holding a dialogue with your "inner child," can be especially helpful in working with your own feelings. There is also a script in the Supplement that can serve as a model for exploring a particular emotion directly. The only technique that will not work is called denial. Feelings don't go away. If you try to ignore them or pretend they aren't there, they tend to become more oppressive. To deal with feelings effectively, you must be prepared to confront and acknowledge them. When you use introspection, always regard your feelings with patience, respect, and compassion. As you explore your inner landscape, keep in mind that strong emotions can often be the result of unmet needs. Make sure you identify these needs, and then take whatever action is necessary to have them met.

In addition to inner explorations, I highly recommend that you seek outside support at this time. It is important to learn about the emotions that accompany breast cancer diagnosis and treatment so that you can stop wondering whether what you are feeling is normal. A woman who is further along in her recovery can be an excellent source of information and reassurance in this area. In addition, there are therapists and counselors who specialize in working with cancer patients and are quite familiar with the range of emotions routinely experienced by women recovering from breast cancer. Support groups are also extremely valuable when you are struggling with unfamiliar, oppressive, or confusing emotions. Being in a breast cancer support group gives you an opportunity to have your feelings heard and validated. As you express your feelings fully, you will find that the weight of them begins to lift. As you participate in a group where these feelings are shared, you will find great comfort in the fact that you are not alone.

EMOTIONAL RERUNS

"it has been three months since my mastectomy," said Frieda, "and in all that time I have not been able to cry."

"You know," I responded, trying to reassure her, "some people think it's abnormal to go through a crisis without crying, but not everyone reacts in the same way. Some women deal with breast cancer without ever shedding a tear. Each person is unique, and it's perfectly okay for you not to cry."

"No, no," she declared, "you don't understand! Sometimes I am so full of sadness that I can actually feel the tears crowding into my throat. There is a terrible weight on my chest, and I know that crying would relieve it. I desperately need to cry, and somehow I just can't seem to let go."

Wondering if there were something in her past that might be blocking her tears, I began to question Frieda about her childhood. She described her early years in Germany, told me about her family, and then mentioned that she had been sent to a concentration camp when she was eleven years old. She had somehow managed to survive until the end of the war, after which she had come to America with her few remaining family members.

"Frieda," I asked, "did you ever cry while you were in the camp?"

"Oh no!" she replied emphatically. "My life depended on holding myself together and keeping my wits about me. If I had cried, I would have lost control, and I would have been unable to protect myself."

Frieda had accurately perceived her experience in the concentration camp as life-threatening and had decided at the time that crying or giving in to her emotions in any way would greatly diminish her chances of staying alive. Tears were a luxury she could not afford. Now her unconscious mind had equated her ordeal in the camp with breast cancer, the most recent threat to her survival. The coping mechanisms that had worked in the earlier crisis were being reactivated, once again preventing her from fully expressing her terror, grief, anger, and sadness. Frieda was experiencing an emotional rerun.

Frequently, a crisis such as breast cancer can put us in touch with potent feelings from the past, especially when those feelings have not been adequately dealt with or resolved. If a woman who is recovering from breast cancer finds that her painful feelings tend to persist, or suspects that she might be overreacting, she may be experiencing an emotional rerun. A rerun is often a signal from the "inner child" that some unfinished business must be attended to. For example, after Frieda was released from the concentration camp, she never really shared her feelings about it with anyone. She wanted to close the door on that part of her life forever. However, her "inner child" had carried around the horror of that experience for over forty years. Frieda had never received the comfort and compassion she so desperately needed. Once she understood why she had been unable to cry, she could choose an appropriate course of action. She decided to join a group for concentration-camp survivors with whom she could share the fear and the loneliness that had been locked up inside her for so long. As the impact of her emotional rerun became clear, Frieda was able to separate the past from the present. It became easier for her to express her feelings, and ultimately she was able to shed the tears she had held back since her breast cancer diagnosis.

As women move through diagnosis, treatment, and recovery from breast cancer, it is normal for them to experience many strong feelings. When these feelings become overwhelming and persist beyond a reasonable length of time, there is a possibility that the current situation is in some way reminiscent of one or several painful experiences from the past. When this happens, the unconscious mind engages in a type of cross-indexing procedure, forging a connection between the old and the new. The feelings that accompanied those old situations are then reactivated. As a result, the emotional reaction to the present crisis is greatly intensified. The feelings grow to unmanageable proportions as a woman is forced to deal with the added burden of old emotional baggage. Unless she understands how the past influences her reactions, she is likely to attribute all her pain to the breast cancer experience.

One day, I received a frantic call from a seventy-two-year-old woman desperately looking for help. Ruth had called the American Cancer Society, only to be told that she had missed the first session of my group. When I lead an eight-week breast cancer group, I prefer to have all participants start together and attend for the full period of time. However, I am always willing to make exceptions when the need arises. The secretary suggested that Ruth get in touch with me directly to see if we could work something out.

"I'm in trouble," she said. "Even though the doctors keep telling me that my cancer has been cured, I have these awful anxiety attacks two or three times a day. I went to a therapist and she referred me to a psychiatrist immediately. He wants to put me on all kinds of pills, including a strong antidepressant. I really don't want to take drugs, but I don't know what else to do. I can't seem to stop crying, and I feel so alone. I know you've already started a group, but do you think I could join even though I've missed some of it? I'm feeling so dreadful, maybe being with other people would help."

I told her that she would be welcome in the group and asked if she would tell me a few things about herself. During our conversation, I found out that Ruth had lost her husband thirteen years earlier. As she told me about it, she began to cry. "If only he were here with me now," she sobbed, "I wouldn't have to go through all this alone." Without realizing it, Ruth had given me the key to her distress. She had been married for many years, and she and her husband had loved each other dearly. His death had left a tremendous emptiness in her life. The protection and comfort she was craving would have been available to her if only he were still alive. Ruth's experience with cancer had stirred up a resurgence of grief over her husband's death. It is not unusual for a breast cancer patient to feel alone. Cancer is a lonely disease. However, Ruth's reaction was only partly due to breast cancer. I explained that the rest of it was coming from another source and would pass if she simply understood it and allowed it to run its course.

Five days later, Ruth arrived promptly for the second session of the group. I introduced her to the other women, and invited her to share her reasons for joining us. She told of her anxiety attacks, her preoccupation with cancer, her reluctance to take any of the medication which had been recommended by the psychiatrist, and her fear that she was becoming emotionally unbalanced. Finally, she told the group about our conversation. "I'm not really sure why," she concluded, "but I haven't had one single anxiety attack since our phone call!" Of course, I was highly gratified, but I was not really surprised. When it comes to emotions, we can cope with reality much more effectively if we are able to separate the past from the present. Ruth continued to attend the group and was very open about her grief over the loss of her husband. Slowly, the strength of her other feelings and concerns began to diminish. In the company of the other group members, she was able to resolve her fears about cancer and to come to terms with the change in her appearance caused by her mastectomy. By the time the group ended, she was full of her customary *joie de vivre* and was planning a monthlong trip to Alaska with her daughter.

During the course of my breast cancer groups, I have heard some women say that they are deeply ashamed of having cancer and of the changes in their bodies. They seem to suffer from a painful sense of differentness, and feel alienated from society. Whenever I encounter this combination of shame and alienation, I tend to suspect that a special kind of emotional rerun is occurring, one related to a dark secret that may have been hidden for many years.

Ernestine was in her mid-forties at the time she attended one of my breast cancer groups. She was shy and reserved and made a special point of letting us know that she was a very private person. She would only say that she had withdrawn from all her friends and acquaintances because of her cancer. She could not believe that anyone would find her acceptable now that she looked so different and had such a "loathsome" disease. She was simply unwilling to face the world, and had even left her job. Knowing that she was in pain, I gave her many opportunities to share her feelings with the rest of the group, but she would always refuse. Clearly, my invitations made her very uncomfortable.

As the group progressed, the women grew more and more supportive of each other. The atmosphere in the room was always very loving and kind. Toward the end of the sixth session, Ernestine must have decided that the group was reasonably safe, because it was then that she finally risked sharing her shameful secret with us. She revealed that she had been gang-raped at the age of twelve. The incident had taken place in the supply closet of her school, and her four attackers were older boys who were also students. When she went home and told her parents about it, they insisted that she must never tell anyone. They refused to call the police because they did not want the family name sullied with such "filth." Ernestine begged to be allowed to stay home from school or, better yet, transfer to another school, but her parents insisted that she conduct herself as if nothing had ever happened. When she returned to school, the word had spread, and Ernestine became an outcast and an object of scorn. Life was very painful for her during the time she was forced to remain in that school.

Eventually, Ernestine graduated, took a secretarial course at the local business school, and moved far away from home. She found a very respectable job, and began to live her life as an independent and self-sufficient adult. She met new people and made several good friends, but she never told anyone about the rape, because she was so ashamed. It had become her dark secret. For so many years, she had just wanted to be like everyone else. This was the one thing in her past that made her feel different. She was convinced that if people knew about it they would reject her. The years passed rather uneventfully until, suddenly, she was diagnosed with breast cancer and had to undergo a mastectomy. Once again she began to feel different from other people, and that feeling stirred up all the pain she had experienced during her teenage years.

When Ernestine finished her recital she sat huddled in her chair, waiting for the other group members to judge, blame, insult, and reject her. What she got instead was fifteen women expressing their sense of outrage at how she had been treated. They assured her that it had not been her fault, and that she had deserved protection, kindness, support, and a family more interested in fighting for her than in protecting themselves. All the women were angry on her behalf and made it clear that she was no less acceptable now than she had been for the past six weeks. In fact, most of the women in the group felt much closer to her now that they knew more about what was going on inside her. At the end of the session, several of the women asked Ernestine to call for reassurance if she began to feel too vulnerable again. When we got together the following week, Ernestine told us that she had been reaching out to her friends once again, and that whenever she started to feel insecure, she would remind herself of the group's reaction. While she still had a great deal of work to do to heal those old wounds, the process had begun in the group. Ernestine no longer had to be burdened by that dark secret of hers, and was beginning to feel free for the first time in many years.

When women carry around shameful secrets, they usually find that life must be limited in some way to guard against exposure. It is amazing how many women decide that past events in their lives make them absolutely unacceptable to others. Much of the time, this is a decision made at such a young age that a person simply does not possess all the necessary information and objectivity to evaluate the event fairly. Once these women have judged themselves as unacceptable, their self-concept is always somewhat damaged, and there are parts of themselves that they cannot feel free to share with others for fear of rejection. When these same women feel safe, supported, and loved, they can finally take advantage of the opportunity to reveal their dark secrets along with the shame which they have endured. The secrets that have been shared in my groups comprise a long and tragic list including rape, incest, physical abuse, desertion by one or both parents, alcoholic parents, imprisonment of a parent, an illegal act that has never been discovered, or a lie that was told sometime in the past. Although I have led countless groups, there has never been a time when these secrets have been received with anything other than kindness and compassion. As difficult as breast cancer is, it can offer women the opportunity to relieve themselves of the ˸urden of shame that they have carried around needlessly for so many years.

Normally, when I lead a breast cancer group, the first three sessions are full of "cancer talk." Women need to share their feelings, compare side effects, discuss treatment alternatives, and deal with serious issues like mortality and recurrence. By the forth session, women are alrcady becoming aware of emotional reruns, and the serious work of healing old wounds usually begins at that time. There are some instances, however, where the connection between the emotional response to a particular aspect of the breast cancer experience and some painful event in the past is not immediately obvious.

Christina had attended one of my eight-week groups and had dealt successfully with many issues, but she was never able to come to terms with her mastectomy. Her boyfriend was very loving and encouraging, telling her that it made no difference to him whatsoever. While Christina was relieved to hear that, it did not alter her own reaction to her body in the slightest. Everytime she looked at herself in a mirror, she would burst into tears. When the group ended, she made an appointment to see me privately so that we could resolve this problem. Sitting in my office, she let me know how discouraged she felt.

"Some of my friends have told me that I must grieve," she said. "They tell me that I should keep crying, because eventually I will cry myself out. Maybe they're right, but there doesn't seem to be an end to my tears. How will I ever get past this?"

"I don't think you are sad and grieving," I replied. "It seems to me that you are really very angry. Will you take a moment and check inside yourself to see if you can find any anger?"

We were silent for a few minutes as she searched within herself. "My goodness!" she said, sounding very surprised. "There's really a ton of anger in there."

"Can you identify the place in your body where that anger is being stored?" I asked.

"Yes," she answered, patting her belly, "it's right here."

I suggested that she close her eyes to see if she could get some visual image of the anger in her belly. "It looks like a huge black cloud," she said.

"Imagine yourself moving into the middle of that cloud, and tell me what it's like in there," I directed.

"It's like a big cave, pretty dark, with a high ceiling. There's something on the far wall, but I can't see it too clearly. Now I'm walking toward it. Oh my God! It's my father's face!"

"Does that have some meaning to you?" I asked.

"It certainly does!" she exclaimed. Then she opened her eyes and told me an incredible story.

When Christina was eight years old, her mother died. Her father was very unhappy to be saddled with the responsibility of raising a little girl and was very vocal about it. He would often ship her off to the homes of various relatives while he pursued some of his academic interests. Christina began to mature early, and by the time she was ten years old she already had fairly well-developed breasts. She was very proud of her breasts and thought they looked beautiful. One day, she overheard a telephone conversation between one of her aunts and her father. Her aunt warned her father not to buy Christina a bra for fear that boys might be attracted to her if she "stuck out." Her father, who was not only busy with his own concerns but very sexually repressed as well, agreed. Several months later the pediatrician discovered that Christina had a curvature of the spine, and recommended that she be put in a brace for a year. Once again her aunt intervened, suggesting that her father refuse any treatment because without it Christina would be less attractive to boys. Once again, her father agreed.

As Christina grew older, the deformity in her spine began to worsen. When her father took her to visit family or friends, he would say, "Christina, bend over and show your curves." Obediently, Christina would hug her shirt tight around her and bend over so that her father could demonstrate how her back curved and her right shoulder blade protruded. As the years went on, Christina used to comfort herself by saying, "I have a lousy back, but my breasts are really nice." Her breasts had become her compensation for having a curvature of the spine.

When Christina turned sixteen, she had had enough of her father's abuse and decided to fight back. She went out and bought herself a sexy French bra. The next time her father said, "Christina, show your curves," she unbuttoned her blouse and showed off her new bra and the breasts she felt so proud of. Her father never made his request again. For years her father had tried not to acknowledge that Christina had become a woman. Now she had finally won.

As she finished her story, Christina said, "As soon as I saw my father's face in the cave, I knew why I have been feeling so much anger. My father never wanted me to have breasts, and now one of them is gone. He has won after all."

Now we both understood why she had been unable to reconcile herself to the loss of her breast. She had been experiencing a massive emotional rerun. For years she had resisted a family conspiracy to deprive her of her sexuality. Unconsciously, she had confused the loss of her breast with her father's many attempts to keep her from becoming a woman. The insight Christina gained about the connection between the present and the past was very important and had an immediate effect on her attitude toward her mastectomy. She was able to separate her anger at her father from her feelings about her body. In a short time her crying stopped and she started to investigate the possibility of breast reconstruction. Once the power of her emotional rerun was fully understood, the healing process could really begin.

It is important to recognize when an emotional rerun is taking place. This insight enables you to gain a better perspective on your emotional reactions to breast cancer and helps you feel more in control. It also calls attention to old wounds, dark secrets, and unfinished business, giving you the opportunity finally to resolve these painful issues from the past. If you cannot seem to get beyond certain feelings during your recovery from breast cancer, ask yourself if there is anything in the present situation that reminds you in some way of an experience in your past. This question alone may be enough to alert you to the presence of an emotional rerun. Even if you are unable to make the connection yourself, don't give up! Sometimes we are too close to a situation to see ourselves objectively. This can be a good time to seek private counseling or to join a support group. At a time when you are feeling vulnerable, confused, and over-whelmed, it is nice to know that help is available, and it is perfectly appropriate to ask for it.

chapter fourteen

LIVING WITH THE FEAR

*m*any women who have had breast cancer say they are very fearful that the disease will recur. They become anxious about physical symptoms and ailments, interpreting every ache or pain as a signal that their cancer has returned. Visits to the doctor for three-month checkups, annual mammograms and chest X rays become an ordeal. Some women report that they begin to panic or become severely depressed several weeks before a doctor's appointment or a lab test actually takes place. Fear of recurrence is entirely normal, especially in the first months following a breast cancer diagnosis. As a woman acquires a track record for normal checkups, her apprehension should begin to fade until it either disappears or reaches a very manageable level. However, when the fear is overwhelming and does not diminish over time, it becomes a problem that must be resolved.

When I ask women specifically why they are afraid of recurrence, they have basically two answers: death itself, and the type of death often associated with cancer. Coming to terms with the idea of death and one's own mortality has been discussed in Chapter 1. I believe that breast cancer does challenge women to develop a better perspective on death. In fact, it is not unusual for people to pursue some form of spiritual growth as a response to confronting their own mortality. However, the idea of dying a prolonged and painful death from cancer is quite another story.

The first time I had breast cancer, I assumed that the treatment had cured me forever. Three-and-a-half years later I found another lump in my breast that also turned out to be malignant. When I first heard the diagnosis, I was in shock . . . then I was frightened . . . and then I was furious! Even though my surgeon had actually told me that there was a chance of a recurrence, I hadn't believed him. I felt as though I had been betrayed by my doctors. After all, I had been a wonderful patient, very cooperative, and almost always pleasant and amusing. As a reward, my medical team was supposed to protect me from cancer and keep me safe. It seemed so unfair that they had let me down.

Once I had run through all these emotions, I settled down to deal with the realities of the situation. My surgeon, Dr. G——, told me that I would need a mastectomy, and then sat quietly with me while I struggled to control a flood of tears. I felt a terrible sense of dread. At that moment, the loss of a breast seemed more catastrophic than the fact that my cancer had recurred. We decided that he would perform the surgery in three weeks. In the meantime, he scheduled me for the many tests that accompany a breast cancer diagnosis: chest X ray, bone scan, blood work, brain scan, mammogram, and liver scan. The purpose of these tests is to determine whether cancer has spread to other areas of the body. I was given an appointment to meet with Dr. G—— once all the tests were completed, so that we could discuss the results. I thought that was a mere formality. It was inconceivable to me that any of the tests could be positive. I had enough to deal with just trying to adjust myself to the fact that I was about to lose my breast.

A week and a half later, on a Friday afternoon, I was sitting in the examination room when Dr. G—— walked in. I looked up, expecting to see his usual warm smile. Instead, he had a strange expression on his face. He looked very serious and very sad. I could feel my heart pounding in my chest as I tried to prepare myself for some bad news. Almost apologetically, he told me that there was some question about my liver scan. That meant there was a possibility that the breast cancer had spread to my liver. He explained that I would need to have another test, called an ultrasound, in order to make a final determination. Since the weekend was coming up, there was no way to schedule me for the ultrasound until the following Monday.

I don't know how I managed to drive home. I felt as though I were encased in a cocoon of terror. When I got to my house, I went straight to my bedroom, took off all my clothes, and got into bed. Shivering uncontrollably, I curled up into a tight ball and huddled under my quilt. All I could think of was that I would die a terrible death in excruciating and unrelenting pain. I could imagine myself becoming totally dependent and gradually wasting away. I felt utterly defenseless. I longed for someone to hold me, to magically protect me from this devastation. I had a terrifying sense of my own aloneness.

I stayed in bed for two whole days, getting up only to drink a little water and to go to the bathroom. I spoke to no one. I had no words—only overwhelming feelings of terror, loneliness, and despair. On Sunday afternoon, I suddenly sat up in bed and I heard myself say, "Wait a minute. Today I'm not in any pain. Chances are that tomorrow won't be that different from today. I really don't know what the future holds, but I know I can take this one day at a time. I know there is a chance that I could die of cancer, and I might have a lot of pain. If ever there comes a time when I feel that the pain is unendurable, I can always kill myself!" As the thought registered, I experienced an immediate sense of relief. The fact that I had it within my power to make this decision gave me back some feeling of control over my own life. I no longer felt like a helpless victim. The problem had been handled. I had found a way to live with the fear. No longer immobilized by my own anxieties, I got out of bed, showered, and went for a walk on the beach. As it turned out, I was lucky. When I went back to the hospital on Monday for the ultrasound, the test showed that my liver was perfectly normal. However, the ordeal that I went through over the weekend has served me well ever since. No one can give me a guarantee that I will never have cancer again. Although I know that I am vulnerable, I no longer worry about dying a long and painful death.

When I tell this story to people who have never had cancer, I get a very mixed reaction. There are those who understand and respond with empathy. Others criticize me for even daring to consider suicide. However, women who are recovering from breast cancer often feel relieved when they hear the story. In all the years that I have been sharing this story with my breast cancer groups, I have never had any group member react negatively. I must hasten to explain that I am not an advocate of suicide. As a psychotherapist, I have worked with many patients who have felt overwhelmed by hopelessness and despair. When things looked bleakest, some of them have considered suicide as a viable alternative to living a pain-filled life. I have always fought hard to help them find a reason to go on living, and to foster a belief in life's untold possibilities. I do believe that, in most cases, emotional pain can be worked through and resolved. However, no amount of psychological insight can relieve the kind of physical pain that we fear may accompany a terminal illness from cancer.

Once I felt as though I had some measure of control over my own death, I began talking to doctors. I found several oncologists who routinely make it clear to their terminally ill patients that they consider pain control to be of primary importance. These doctors explain that they do whatever is necessary to control the level of pain. They will frequently give their patients the opportunity to choose between pain and consciousness. If a patient wants to remain conscious, she might have to be willing to tolerate greater discomfort. If she wishes to reduce the level of pain, she could agree to have more medication in exchange for less consciousness. The important point is, what had once been a private terror and a matter of the gravest concern to the patient has now become a subject which can be dealt with cooperatively by a woman and her doctor.

There are some women who tell me that they cannot seem to escape the fear of recurrence. It colors every waking moment and haunts their dreams. I will sometimes ask my groups to imagine the hypothetical case of a forty-five-year-old woman who has just been treated for cancer. She lives the next fifty years totally paralyzed by the fear of recurrence, only to die of a heart attack at the age of ninety-five. Fifty terror-filled, unproductive years. What an incredible waste! It is vitally important to allow yourself to reinvest in life so that this very precious gift will not be wasted. We have all been vulnerable from the day of our birth. That is simply a fact of the human condition. Cancer only puts a convenient and concrete label on this state of vulnerability. One could just as easily step off a curb on the way to the supermarket and be hit by a bus, although few of us lose much sleep worrying about that.

Offering a woman a change of perspective or a philosophical base from which to view her situation does not always resolve the fear of recurrence. Sometimes, a deeper kind of work needs to be done so that the underlying cause of this persistent fear can be understood. For example, some women are convinced that cancer is a punishment for a past transgression. In order to alleviate the fear of recurrence, these women must be helped to resolve guilty feelings of long standing. In such cases, counseling, either with a psychotherapist or a religious adviser, can be very effective.

There are also times when a woman's focus on breast cancer may actually obscure the real cause of her emotional distress. One woman contacted me a year after she had "graduated" from one of my breast cancer groups to tell me that her fear of recurrence had suddenly returned and she was experiencing considerable anxiety and depression. I asked her to come to my office for a private session so that we could do some detective work. As we talked about her life, she disclosed that she was approaching her fiftieth birthday and still had no goals. She was going through a delayed mid-life crisis and was beginning to panic because she had no real direction in life. I pointed out that it wasn't really cancer that she feared at all. She was afraid that her life would be over before she was able to accomplish anything of significance. Once the problem was clearly defined, we were able to resolve it in rather short order.

A certain percentage of women do have to deal with an actual recurrence of breast cancer. A few have told me that it is easier the second time because they know what to expect, but most women are far more frightened the second time. They wonder whether the treatment they received the first time had any effect at all. They often feel discouraged and hopeless. However, they soon mobilize themselves and begin once again to fight for their lives. It is important to understand that while a recurrence is a serious situation, it is by no means an automatic death sentence. For some women, a recurrence is a fairly simple affair which requires short-term treatment and marks the end of any further evidence of the disease. For others, cancer may become a chronic illness. In such cases, treatment may be needed periodically, but women are still able to enjoy a good quality of life and can survive for many years. Once again, the crucial issue is whether a woman can overcome her fear of recurrence sufficiently to enjoy the remainder of her life.

Emily was sixty-four at the time she attended one of my breast cancer workshops. She was a small, slender, silver-haired woman who seemed very timid and shy. She had been treated for breast cancer twenty years before and had just experienced a recurrence. During the course of the daylong workshop, she was able to express some of her feelings, especially her fear and her difficulty with body image. When the day was over, she mentioned that it had been very comforting to hear her particular concerns echoed by so many other women. Before leaving, she asked if she could see me privately. I told her that would be fine and handed her my card. That was the last I heard of her for four months.

When she did call, she apologized for the delay. The idea of therapy had made her very nervous, although the workshop had brought up several issues that needed attention. It had taken her a while to admit to herself that they were problems she really couldn't handle alone. As we began to work, it became clear that only a few of her concerns were directly related to breast cancer. Many of her other fears had to do with a very difficult childhood that had resulted in her conviction that the world was a dangerous place. Slowly we addressed one old wound after another, giving her "inner child" a chance finally to be heard. Gradually, Emily started to feel less fearful and more self-confident. She was pleased with her progress, and often came to a session reporting some victory in an area that had previously caused her considerable distress.

We had been working together for about six months when Emily phoned to tell me that her doctor had discovered a tumor in her neck that turned out to be malignant. Her cancer had spread to a lymph node in her neck, and tests showed that it had also metastasized to her liver. Needless to say, when Emily came in for her next session, she was terrified. She was scheduled to begin radiation immediately, after which her doctor prescribed an indefinite course of chemotherapy. As the weeks wore on, Emily reported that she was experiencing extreme anxiety along with a debilitating depression. Although she was not in pain, she was so consumed with fear that she couldn't enjoy even a single moment of any day. She either slept or trembled. Her husband tried to provide diversions, but she was unable to focus on anything except her disease. To make matters worse, she was also furious at herself for wasting what time she had.

To counteract some of her anxiety, I began teaching Emily some basic relaxation techniques. They helped a little, but it was obvious that there was much more work to be done. I suggested that guided imagery might be very useful in helping her confront and resolve some of her worst fears. This was not at all what she wanted to hear. Her choice had been to run from her fears rather than to confront them. Her very worst fear was that death was actively pursuing her. Because her methods of coping had not worked, Emily agreed, with considerable trepidation, to try mine.

I asked her to sit back in her chair, close her eyes, and allow an image to form itself in her mind. Once she had an image, she was to describe to me what she saw.

"I see Death," she said, her voice filled with panic.

"What does Death look like?" I asked.

"She is a tall woman in a dark cape. Her eyes are black and intense. Her face is very thin and drawn. She looks almost like a skeleton. Now she is starting to walk toward me with her arms outstretched. Her fingers are long and bony, and her hands are beginning to curl like claws. She is reaching for me. I can't escape. Help me! I'm so frightened."

"Emily," I said, "I want you to tell her that she is frightening you. Ask her if she will agree to stand still for a while so that you can talk to her."

After a few moments, Emily continued, "She stopped. She said she didn't realize that she was scaring me. I begged her for more time. Death explained that she was helpless. She told me that I had to accept the fact that she exists, but the rest was up to me. After that, she started to change. She got smaller and less threatening and I could see that she was looking sad. I think she was sorry she had to be there at all. Finally, she began to recéde into the background until she disappeared."

"Did you understand what Death meant when she said that the rest is up to you?" I asked.

"Oh yes," said Emily. "She was telling me that I can choose to keep her in the background so that I can live my life now."

The following week, Emily said that she had noticed a slight improvement. Waking up in the morning, however, was still terrible. She was feeling overwhelmed with anxiety until around four o'clock in the afternoon. As evening approached, she would start feeling better, only to have the same cycle begin all over again the next day. Her husband told her that from morning to night she was like two entirely different people. On a hunch, I asked her how old she felt when she woke up in the morning.

"I feel like a first-grader," she replied. "When I was in first grade, I had a teacher named Mrs. Smith. She was very cruel, and always embarrassed me in front of the other children. On school days, I used to lie in bed, filled with dread, hoping I could convince my mother that I was sick. Usually, my mother didn't believe me, so I would have to get up, go to school and face that terrible dragon."

"It seems that you had a real live dragon waiting for you out there when you were a child," I said. "Now cancer probably feels like the dragon. When you open your eyes in the morning, the first thing you must think of is that cancer is waiting to grab you and hurt you."

Surprised, Emily said, "Why, yes, that is exactly what it feels like!"

I asked her if she would like to get rid of that dragon once and for all. When she nodded, I suggested that she close her eyes and allow an image of the dragon to form in her mind. Once Emily let me know that she had a clear picture of the dragon, I suggested that she had the power to conjure up all the tools she would need to help her destroy the beast.

"What a huge dragon he is," Emily said, as she began to describe the scene. "He looks terribly vicious, and he breathes fire. I don't know how I could kill him."

"Perhaps you could start by dismantling him," I suggested.

"Yes," she said, "that would work. First, I'll chop off his tail. Now I can push the tail off the hill we're standing on, and into the tar pit below. Good! The tail has disappeared into the tar pit. Uh-oh, now he's starting to tilt forward and his head is getting lower. That's very scary."

I encouraged her to stay a safe distance from the head. "What else could you do in the meantime?" I asked.

"I could saw off the bumps on his back," she replied. "Okay, that's done. I have just pushed that whole part of him off the hill and into the tar pit. It threw the dragon off balance, and he fell over. His head is still very threatening, so I had better stay away from it. I know what I can do next. I can unscrew his legs. Now he can't move at all!"

Once Emily had immobilized the dragon, I felt that she was prepared to face his head. I suggested that she stand a safe distance away and imagine herself roaring at the dragon. Gradually, her posture and her breathing began to change. Finally, she said in an angry voice, "I feel like smashing his head in with a club!" After she had done so, she proceeded to saw off the head and shove it into the tar pit as well.

"What about the rest of the dragon?" I asked her.

"I can just leave it," she said. "There's not enough there to scare me."

"Are you ready to return to this room yet?"

Emily grinned. "I have one more thing to do. I am making a sign that says, 'I killed this dragon. Do not disturb.' "

It is now six months later. I am pleased to report that Emily is responding well to chemotherapy. She and her husband have been enjoying the simple pleasures of life on a daily basis. Emily tells me that she gets a jolt of fear every now and then, especially when she has a doctor's appointment, but it dissipates quickly. She is feeling very proud of herself for taking charge of her life and conquering many of her fears. When people ask her, in amazement, how she can be doing so well when her state of health is so precarious, she smiles and says, "First you kill your dragon, and then you go ahead and live life."

chapter fifteen

———————— □ ————————

THE IMPORTANCE
OF GOOD
COMMUNICATION

*d*uring an experience with breast cancer, it is normal to feel the need for comfort, support, validation, and empathy. Women look to family and friends, expecting those people with whom they are most closely connected to come through for them in a crisis situation. However, many of the women who have attended my groups report feelings of disappointment, frustration, sadness, anger, or despair when they find that their needs are not being met. It is not unusual to find some basic difficulties in communication at the root of these problems.

When I had my first surgery for breast cancer, I was often angry, disappointed, or deeply hurt by the reactions from people I knew. There were a few who never called. I didn't hear from them for months. Later, I found out that they didn't know what to say and were afraid that they might upset me. Some people who did reach me managed to say exactly the wrong things. One woman burst into my room the day after my operation and exclaimed, "Thank God you didn't have to lose your breast!" I was stunned. "How can she be thinking about my breast," I wondered, "when I have just been told that I have this awful disease that may cost me my life?"

The entire time I was in the hospital, I never felt that there was any respect for my privacy. Two days after surgery, I was still on strong pain medication. I looked dreadful, and I felt worse. The last thing I wanted was company. Unfortunately, it happened to be Sunday, a day when people have the leisure to attend to their "obligations." By two o'clock in the afternoon, my room was filled with fifteen well-meaning visitors, most of whom were just acquaintances. I was exhausted, my hair was a mess, my arm was hurting me, and I hadn't the strength to put on any makeup. I felt unkempt, exposed, embarrassed, and trapped. It never occurred to me to ask them to leave. After all, I had been brought up to be considerate, and my manners were beyond reproach. Good manners notwithstanding, I found myself stockpiling a great deal of anger and resentment.

Months later, I began to review my reactions to these events. In retrospect, I saw that much of the responsibility had been mine. I had systematically avoided any opportunity to communicate my needs. There were times when I did not have a clear idea of what my needs were. I was often concerned that expressing my needs would seem rude, inappropriate, or burdensome, and I was unwilling to risk insulting people or making them feel uncomfortable. I realized that there were situations where I was waiting for other people to read my mind, having always believed that if someone really cared about me, he (she) would know what I wanted without my ever saying anything. I was finally able to admit that depending on others to guess my needs was useless and self-defeating. I came to the conclusion that people don't usually say or do hurtful things deliberately. They might just be feeling awkward or uncomfortable. In difficult and emotion-filled situations, a surprising number of people are completely unaware of how to be supportive or helpful.

During the next three years, I taught myself a great deal about communication. I came to understand that communication always involves both a sender and a receiver. In the past, when my needs had not been met, I had blamed the receiver. I was beginning to appreciate that, as the sender, it was my responsibility to convey my own needs and wants to others in a clear, direct, nonthreatening way. I learned how to sit quietly and listen for messages from my "inner child" that would clarify what my needs really were. I gave myself permission to be honest and open about my feelings. I learned to put my own needs first without feeling guilty.

The second time I faced a breast cancer diagnosis, I was determined not to make the same mistakes. When I thought of the difficult time that lay ahead, I knew exactly what I would need, and I took action immediately. One by one, I called all my relatives in New York— aunts, uncles, and cousins, as well as my immediate family. "I'm going through a difficult time," I said, "and I need your help. I just found out that I have breast cancer again. I am terribly frightened, and I feel very alone. What I need most of all is a phone call once a week. When you call, I would like you to tell me that my being alive has mattered to you in some way. I need to know that our connection is important to you." Not a day went by without at least one phone call from someone in my family. Each of the calls was unique and very precious, reminding me again and again how very much I was loved. Even though the reality of my medical situation hadn't changed, those phone calls made me feel much more secure. I had learned that the best way to get what I needed was to ask for it. Once my family knew exactly what I wanted, they were only too happy to oblige.

Assuming that a woman knows what she needs, she must then be willing to ask for it. I often find that the women in my breast cancer groups have difficulty communicating their needs to others. This is especially true when a woman has fallen prey to the super-woman syndrome. Many women are convinced that they must be all things to all people all the time, no matter what! The burdens they carry are enormous. They demand perfection of themselves in many areas. They set unrealistic standards and then struggle to live up to them. Best wife, most nurturing mother, most productive and dependable employee . . . the list goes on and on. These are the women who are always helping others but are unable to accept any help themselves. The problem is that when a superwoman gets breast cancer, she is just as frightened and feels just as fragile as anyone else. Rather than asking for comfort or support, she tries to take care of herself and everyone else in her world. She takes on these responsibilities at a time when she is least able to deal with them.

Eventually, she winds up feeling exhausted, discouraged, and depressed.

Laura came to one of my groups four months after she had been diagnosed with breast cancer. She was undergoing chemotherapy and was having a very difficult time. Her energy level was extremely low, she felt quite ill, and after a treatment she would be nauseated for long periods of time. However, it was not her reaction to chemotherapy that troubled her. Laura had two teenagers at home, and she was very anxious to have family life go on as usual. The sicker she felt, the more determined she was to act the part of the healthy, competent, energetic mother. She told the group that she was plagued by terrible guilt and depression because she found herself unable to meet all her children's demands. Under normal circumstances, there would have been nothing unusual about these demands, which involved a considerable amount of shopping and chauffeuring, combined with various unscheduled minor emergencies. However, these were not normal circumstances. Laura was unwilling to admit to the children that she simply could not handle the job alone and desperately needed their help.

The group asked Laura why she was clinging so tenaciously to her role as superwoman. She explained that the children's father had died of cancer six years before. It had been a very difficult time for the whole family. At the time, Laura had sworn that she would devote herself to making her children feel secure. A few years later, she remarried. Her second husband was a kind and loving man, and the children seemed very happy with their new stepfather. Life moved along peacefully until Laura was diagnosed with breast cancer. Suddenly her world was turned upside down. Now Laura was trying desperately to protect her children from the fear that they would lose her to cancer the same way they had lost their father. She believed that if she could somehow carry on as usual, her children would assume that she could not be seriously ill, and they would not worry that she might die.

It took the group a while to convince Laura that what she was doing was counterproductive. It was clear that her body was making urgent demands for rest, and those demands had to be respected. In addition, her children were already very familiar with the seriousness of a cancer diagnosis. The only thing Laura's superwoman act accomplished was to keep her children from discussing the situation with her. Instead, everyone was trying to pretend that things were okay, and no one really believed it. We pointed out that she could be far more helpful to her children if she were to encourage open communication, listening to their feelings, answering their questions, and telling them specifically what kind of help she needed from them. Laura agreed and decided to talk to her children the next day. When she returned to group the following week, she looked happier and much more relaxed. She and her children had spent a great deal of time together. They had cried together and hugged a lot. Once the truth had been told and good communication had been established, Laura found that the children were very willing to assume a share of the household chores and errands. Within a short time, she was able to retire from her position as resident superwoman and allow herself to be a real person. She learned what so many superwomen need to discover: it is sometimes just as important to receive as it is to give.

Laura's story brings up an important point about telling the truth. Sometimes we think we are doing other people a service when we try to shield them from the truth. Actually, this kind of protection often causes a great deal of harm. It sends an indirect message to people, telling them that they are not strong enough to cope with life's realities. Withholding the truth is the best way to cripple our children and teach them to fear life. It tends to create confusion, misunderstanding, and distance between people, and often causes feelings of alienation and mistrust.

Last year, I ran a support group for the daughters of women with breast cancer. The problems that came up most frequently had to do with the secrecy surrounding a mother's illness. Karen, a thirty-six-year-old mother of three, was sixteen when her own mother was first treated for breast cancer. Although her mother was seriously ill, her father kept insisting that there was nothing wrong. Sometimes her mother would cry and say that she was afraid of dying. When Karen asked her father about it, he would reply that her mother was hysterical and that Karen would do well to ignore her. Because her father was a very powerful and convincing man, Karen had no real reason to doubt him. She began to suspect that her mother might be having some kind of emotional breakdown. She did not realize that, because she was the "baby" of the family, her father had been trying to protect her.

Having been assured repeatedly that all was well, Karen was out of town the day that her mother died. When Karen was told that her mother had passed away, she went into shock. She had been completely unprepared. Once the shock wore off, grief and anger took its place. She had been cheated out of all the time that she might have spent being close to her mother. She felt manipulated and betrayed by her father. Worst of all, she suffered terrible guilt. How could she forgive herself for not being there to comfort her mother in those last days? How could she have let her mother die alone? Feeling a deep sense of shame, Karen became convinced that she was a selfish and thoughtless person. She carried the pain of this experience with her for twenty years until she was finally able to resolve the matter in therapy. Ironically, her father's efforts to protect Karen from grief, loss, and fear had exactly the opposite effect. What she had really needed was help in facing the truth and permission to express her feelings fully.

Most women who go through a breast cancer experience find that there are times when they really need to share their feelings with others. They want to have their feelings heard by someone who is capable of being a good and compassionate listener. Unfortunately, good listeners are sometimes hard to find. What characteristics make a good listener? The best explanation I have ever heard came from a twenty-eight-year-old woman named Courtney. She had been a private patient of mine for two years and had made great strides in her own personal development. One day, she entered my office for her appointment and immediately began to cry. It seems that, when she was sixteen, she had lost all but peripheral vision in her right eye. Her doctors gave her every reason to believe that the other eye would remain normal. Several days before her appointment, the vision in her good eye began to blur. Courtney was terrified that she might be going blind. She wept and she raged; she demanded an answer to the eternal question "Why me?" She cursed God, and she declared that all her work in therapy had been in vain. Once she was able to express her feelings, Courtney gradually grew calmer and more in control of herself, until, finally, she was able to discuss plans and alternatives. Before she left my office, I asked her what she had wanted from me that day. She said, "I needed you to *stay in the room* and to *understand*."

There are many ways for a listener to "leave the room." The most obvious is to simply get up and walk out. The more subtle ways include interrupting, trying to change the subject, telling a person that she shouldn't feel the way she feels, advising, solving, judging, and criticizing. An interaction with this kind of listener will often leave a woman feeling misunderstood, frustrated, unsupported, rejected, and very lonely. It is important to understand that what keeps a person from "staying in the room" may have nothing to do with impatience, disinterest, or disapproval but rather with fear—the fear of not being able to solve the problem and heal the pain. A listener will often struggle to find solutions when there really are none, just to avoid confronting his own powerlessness. If there are no solutions, then the listener may try to escape.

Not too long ago, I got a call from a friend in New York. Gail knew that I worked with cancer patients and that I had been a cancer patient myself. She had a problem and thought I might be able to help.

"My friend Phyllis is terminally ill," she said. "She has been in and out of the hospital constantly for the last three months. Yesterday, she felt well enough to go out to lunch, so I took her to the country club. We were sitting at the table with some of the other women she knows, when someone brought up the subject of a dinner dance that was going to take place in six months. In a perfectly normal voice, Phyllis said, 'Who knows if I'll even be here by then.' There was a dreadful silence at the table, and then a flurry of meaningless conversation. I felt terrible. Phyllis shared something important, and it just got ignored. I felt so awkward, I didn't know what to do. What should I have said?"

"What did you want to say to her?" I asked.

"I had this urge to say, 'Don't worry, Phyllis. You'll be here. I promise!' "

"Well, I can understand the urge, but it's a promise you could never keep, and you would both know it." I thought for a moment, trying to put myself in Phyllis's place, and then said, "I still believe that the truth is the best way to go. I would say, 'Phyllis, I don't know whether you'll be here in six months, but I'm so glad you're here now. You're a wonderful friend and I love you very much.' "

Gail went over to Phyllis's house the next day and said basically what I had suggested. The next time she called, she told me that they had spent a most wonderful and loving time together, freed from all pretenses and able to be real with each other. Two weeks later Phyllis died. Gail was grateful that she had been able to reach out—not only for Phyllis's sake, but for her own as well. By being willing to "stay in the room" rather than find a solution or run away, she had been able to experience a truly extraordinary level of closeness with another human being.

It is impossible for two people to connect when one is trying to communicate feelings and the other is determined to search for practical solutions. In those cases, both parties wind up feeling frustrated and misunderstood. Actually, being heard *is* the solution. It relieves the pressure of the emotions that may have been building up for days or weeks, it helps us to feel connected to others in a very important way, and it takes away some of the loneliness.

Once you are able to recognize problems in communication, you can take steps to resolve them. Ask yourself whether you are being clear about your needs and your feelings. If the answer is no, you may need to spend some time learning how to be more direct. Sometimes it may be necessary to educate the people in your life so that they can become better listeners. They need to know that being heard and understood makes you feel better; that crying is not a problem but a release, and your tears should be allowed to run their course; that your feelings need to be heard and not solved; and that the greatest gift they can give you is to "stay in the room." Good communication is important. Human beings were not designed to live in a vacuum. We rely on each other for support and encouragement. As we establish better, more effective, communication with the people in our life, we will find that they can contribute in very significant ways to our emotional healing.

chapter sixteen

TAKING BACK POWER

*i*rene was fifty-two at the time of her breast cancer diagnosis. She had undergone a lumpectomy and was just finishing her radiation therapy when she joined one of my eight-week support groups. Her overriding concerns had to do with the fear of recurrence and death. During the first few sessions, she was very tearful and spoke at length about her anxieties. By the time five weeks had gone by, Irene was much calmer and happier. She had benefited greatly from being able to share her feelings with the group and had been comforted by the fact that other women felt as she did. Confident that she had taken some major steps toward emotional recovery, I was shocked to see how depressed and hopeless she looked when she arrived for the sixth session. When I asked what had happened, she told a very disturbing story.

"I have been examining my breasts once a month for the past ten years," she said. "I was the one who found the lump in my breast that turned out to be cancer. I felt good about that. I felt that my diligence had been rewarded because the doctor said it was caught early and I had a very good chance of being cured. Last week, I found a lump in my other breast. I panicked, called my doctor's office, and set up an appointment. When I went in, he examined me and found nothing. He told me that it is pretty common for women to react this way after they have had breast cancer, and that I should go home, have a glass of wine, and relax. I know my body. I know there's a lump because I can still feel it. He doesn't believe me, and there's nothing I can do. I guess I'm going to die."

Irene felt powerless. Her life was at stake, and she had no idea how to fight for it. She was a member of a health maintenance organization (HMO), and did not have the money to go elsewhere to seek a second opinion. Even though she was aware that she could request another doctor within the group, she believed that it would be hopeless because she would already have been branded a hysterical female, and her credibility would have been totally compromised. As her feelings of powerlessness increased, so did her depression, until she was completely immobilized.

Irene had to be convinced that she had certain rights as a patient, and then she needed help figuring out what her options were. Once a course of action was decided upon, the group provided her with a speech that she could practice at home. She was instructed to make an appointment with the administrator of her HMO and tell him the following:

"I'm having a problem. Three months ago, I found a lump in my breast, and I was diagnosed and treated for breast cancer. Last week, I found a lump in my other breast. The doctor who examined me couldn't find the lump, and told me that my imagination has been working overtime. I examine my breasts monthly, and I know that I'm right. I want you to assign a new doctor to my case immediately. I need someone who will examine me without any bias, find the lump, and biopsy it. Otherwise, I will go to a private physician, even if it means putting myself in debt. I have no doubt that he will find the lump in my breast. If that should happen, then I'm going to sue this organization—and I will do it as publicly as possible."

The next day, Irene did exactly as the group had suggested. Within fifteen minutes after her meeting with the administrator, another doctor examined her and found the lump. She had a biopsy the same day and came to the group the following week to report a double victory. Not only had she been heard and validated, but, in addition, the lump turned out to be benign.

While Irene's story is very dramatic, her underlying feelings of powerlessness are shared by many women as they move through an experience with breast cancer. If problems should arise in the doctor-patient relationship, women often feel intimidated and out of control. Many of us have been brought up with the belief that doctors are all-powerful and all-knowing and must therefore be respected and obeyed without question. We are expected to feel grateful for the care we get, even if that care is in some way inadequate. When something occurs that feels wrong, we would rather relinquish our own power than run the risk of alienating the very people we are counting on to save our lives. It is vitally important that women who are dealing with breast cancer be encouraged to act in such a way that they take back their power and achieve some sense of control. In particular, they must be able to deal with their doctors in a straightforward manner. To that end, I have compiled a list of the twelve "rights" most often focused on by the women in my breast cancer groups.

A Patient's Bill of Rights

1. You have the right to be active in your own health care.
2. You have the right to ask questions and to receive understandable answers to those questions.
3. You have the right to say you don't understand and to have something clarified.
4. You have the right to a second opinion.
5. You have the right to be heard and taken seriously.
6. You have the right to be treated with respect and kindness by your health-care providers.
7. You have the right to ask about treatment plans, medications, side effects, and alternatives *before* you give your approval or consent for anything.
8. You have the right to have your phone calls returned promptly.

9. You have the right to be told the truth.
10. You have the right to be fully informed as to the cost of treatment.
11. You have the right to communicate when something happens that you don't like, so that you and your doctor can reach some agreement about a more productive way of dealing with each other.
12. You have the right to change doctors if you are not satisfied with the care you have been receiving.

I do not mean to imply that all doctors are insensitive or psychologically unaware. Many of the women who come to my groups feel fortunate to have doctors who are not only highly competent but kind and caring as well. These women find their relationship with their doctor to be an important source of support and reassurance which often continues even after treatment has ended.

Sometimes, if a doctor-patient relationship is unsatisfactory, it may take just a simple communication to set it right. One group member used the Patient's Bill of Rights to assess her relationship with her doctor and came to the conclusion that she deserved something more. The next time she had an appointment with her oncologist, she said, "Doctor, this is the last time I'll be seeing you, and I want to tell you why. Every time I come in, you spend three minutes with me, tell me that I'm fine, and then you leave. You're always in a hurry. You never ask me if I have any questions, and you never ask me how I'm doing emotionally. I feel as though you couldn't care less about me, and I've begun to resent that. I still have four months of chemotherapy left, and I want to be in treatment with someone who sees me as a person rather than just a cancer patient. I need to be able to count on his undivided attention during my appointment, no matter how busy he is. I have no doubt that you have given me the best medical care, but I want a doctor who will relate to me differently." Much to her surprise, the doctor sat down, thanked her sincerely for the feedback, and spent half an hour with her. In that short time, the basis for a much warmer and more personal relationship was established. Needless to say, the woman stayed with her doctor and was delighted with the change.

Aside from the doctor-patient relationship, women who are dealing with breast cancer are confronted by many other situations that can evoke feelings of powerlessness. Doreen was sixty-two at the time of her mastectomy. Until then, she had been working as a secretary for a major corporation. After surgery, her doctor put her on disability for four months to ensure that her physical recovery would be complete before she had to return to work. By the time Doreen came to a group session, she had three weeks of disability left. She was having trouble sleeping at night and was plagued by frequent bouts of weeping. The idea of going back to work was making her feel exceedingly tense and anxious. Being a very shy and private person, she had not told anyone at work that she had been treated for breast cancer. Of course, they all knew that she was out on sick leave, but no one knew exactly why. Doreen was worried that she would be surrounded by a huge group of co-workers, some of them well-meaning, many of them simply curious, all pressing her for details. She was convinced that if anyone knew about her illness, they would treat her differently. She was already beginning to feel very self-conscious, imagining that everyone would be staring at her chest, trying to figure out which breast she had lost. Doreen felt powerless to resist answering the questions that she knew were inevitable.

It wasn't cancer that made Doreen feel powerless. She had felt powerless, especially in her dealings with other people, for most of her life. However, it was a cancer-related situation that was forcing her to confront this long-standing issue. Doreen had been raised in a very traditional home. As a daughter, she was taught to be sweet, understanding, supportive, nurturing, helpful, accommodating, and most of all, obedient. Power and assertiveness were reserved for the males in the family. No one ever told her that, as an adult, she had the right to privacy. It never occurred to her that she could refuse to answer questions without any apologies or explanations. Once she understood the basis for her feelings of powerlessness and the importance of seeing herself as an equal rather than a subordinate, the group gave her a formula to use when she went back to work. If anyone approached her with a question about the reason for her absence, she was to say, "I would really prefer not to discuss it. Thank you for asking, and I'm feeling fine now." In the event that someone might be tactless enough to persist, Doreen was instructed to simply repeat the first sentence as many times as necessary. She returned to her job a few weeks later. Much to her amazement, her co-workers heard what she had to say and were very respectful of her privacy.

A very interesting phenomenon occurs when the women in my groups begin to address the issue of powerlessness. At first, they consider the problem only in relation to cancer. Very soon, however, it becomes clear that what they are learning is applicable to every area of life. If they have always been accustomed to pleasing others, they now learn to consider their own needs and to say no without guilt. They learn to think of themselves as important and to take themselves seriously. As they gain in self-respect, their sense of power increases. As they come to the conclusion that they deserve to be treated well, they become willing to deal with others much more assertively and to communicate their needs and feelings honestly without fear of reprisal. One by one, they bring in stories to share with the group—stories of small victories in everyday life, each one marking a major shift in self-concept and a tremendous enhancement of personal power.

There are times during the breast cancer experience when even the most powerful of women may be so immobilized by fear or so debilitated by treatment that they cannot stand up for themselves. Marla, a highly respected professor at a major university, was forty at the time of her mastectomy. She was accustomed to dealing with situations competently and assertively and was never intimidated by other people. Although she was finding chemotherapy extremely difficult, Marla was still working full time and handling all the responsibilities of home and family as well. During the time she attended one of my eight-week groups, her major concern was her adverse reaction to chemotherapy. Unfortunately, the side effects she experienced were severe. Nausea had been a continuing problem, and her energy level had been extremely low for several weeks. As treatment progressed, she began to feel more exhausted and fragile with each passing day.

One evening she arrived at group looking white and shaken. "I think I need some help," she said. "Today I went out to buy my prosthesis. I was feeling awkward and uncomfortable about it right from the start. The only people who have seen me without my breast so far are my doctors and my husband. The idea of taking my shirt off for someone I didn't even know was pretty distressing, but I kept telling myself that these women are specialists, and they must know what they're doing. The saleswoman who waited on me seemed very sure of herself. She kept pushing me to make a decision, but I had a lot of questions. Suddenly, she started to yell at me, told me I was wasting her time, and stormed out of the dressing room. Everyone in the shop could hear her. I felt so humiliated, it was all I could do to collect myself and get out of there. I made it to my car just in the nick of time. It was ten minutes before I could stop crying and drive home. I feel abused and angry, but what bothers me the most is how I feel about myself. Normally, I would never let anyone do something like that to me. I would have spoken up for myself immediately. I don't know what happened, but I just couldn't seem to say anything at all. Now, I just feel weak and useless. I know I should do something about this, but I don't know what, and I'm not sure I could even go back there."

Marla had always perceived herself as a powerful person, and now she was feeling as though she had lost an essential part of herself. I hastened to reassure her that this state of powerlessness was temporary, and that when her treatment was over, she would find herself functioning just as she had before her breast cancer diagnosis. It was important that she use what little energy she had for getting through the rest of chemotherapy. In order to deal with the situation at hand, she would have to borrow power from someone else. As it happens, her husband, Jeff, was the perfect candidate. Jeff was already angry that cancer had dared to attack his wife and threaten his home and family. He was constantly feeling frustrated because he couldn't find a target for all that anger. It was easy for Marla to imagine how delighted Jeff would be to intervene on her behalf.

When she returned home after the session, Marla discussed the situation with Jeff. He assured her that he was willing to help in any way she wished. Together they considered several alternatives, including going back to the shop and having Jeff speak to the owner while Marla stood behind him, or even having Marla talk while Jeff stood behind her. Ultimately, Marla decided that she would be most comfortable composing a strong letter, because then she could be sure that everything she wanted to say would be communicated. With Jeff's help, she soon drafted and mailed a letter. The owner of the shop responded immediately, calling to say how sorry she was that Marla had been treated so poorly and assuring her that measures were being taken to see that nothing like that ever happened again. By the time Marla returned to the group the following week, the problem had been handled, and her sense of personal power had been restored.

Having breast cancer is hard. Women are suddenly catapulted into dangerous and unfamiliar territory. We must deal with doctors, nurses, and technicians we have never met before. We must undergo a myriad of tests and procedures, struggle with medical terminology, cope with hospitals and surgery, and tolerate treatments that can range from unpleasant to devastating. We must come to terms with our own mortality and master fear, despair, loneliness, grief, and rage. Given this many challenges, is it any wonder that we are awash in feelings of powerlessness? Taking back power is a learning process that occurs on many levels. It involves gathering as much information as possible about the situation you are in, becoming familiar with your inner feelings, and communicating honestly and directly with others. It requires reaching out to others for help and support and looking inward to discover your own personal strengths. It demands a willingness to face difficult truths and come to terms with them. As you take back power, you will find that you are no longer a cancer "victim." Instead, you will be able to enjoy a sense of mastery and a feeling of accomplishment as you take an active part in your own emotional recovery from breast cancer.

AFTERWORD

CRISIS: A NEW PERSPECTIVE

The Chinese character for crisis is a combination of two words: danger and opportunity. When a woman is first diagnosed with breast cancer, the dangers are obvious. At that moment, it is difficult to imagine that anything beneficial could ever come from such a cataclysmic event. The true challenge of breast cancer is to recognize the importance of the crisis and to be able to use the experience in a positive way, extracting from it what you have learned and applying those lessons to every area of your life.

The benefit of coming to terms with mortality lies not only in reducing the anxiety relating to breast cancer but in helping to change your perspective on life in general. When you learn to understand your deepest feelings and take care of your "inner child," you become a more complete and compassionate human being. As your ability to communicate improves, so will your relationships with people, helping you to feel more powerful and more connected to others, no matter what the situation. If, through an experience with breast cancer, you must confront issues of low self-esteem and negative self-image, the resolution of these issues will remain with you throughout your life. To make breast cancer meaningful, you must be willing to use it as a springboard for personal growth. As you move past the danger and take full advantage of the opportunities hidden within the crisis, you will find that you are better prepared to face any challenge that life may bring.

Touch me—I'm like you
    A hungry soul seeking
    to rediscover
    soft innocence forgotten
    under age's hard cover.

Touch me—I'm like you
    A loving soul seeking
    to share
    our sameness and difference,
    our delight and our despair.

Touch me—I'm like you
    A wounded soul seeking
    to set free
    the grace, the dignity,
    and the courage just to be.

Touch me—I'm like you
    A boundless soul forever seeking
    to bind
    the wonder of existence
    to the relentless passage of time.

                    Anonymous

RELAXATION
AND
IMAGERY

DEEP RELAXATION

*M*ost imagery work begins with some form of relaxation. The value of achieving a state of deep relaxation is that it enables people to get in touch with the creative, image-producing part of their brain more efficiently. As with any new behavior, relaxation techniques must be learned. This learning takes place through repeated practice sessions. As the process becomes more familiar, most people find that they are able to reach a deep level of relaxation in a fairly short time.

In this section, you will find a "script" to use that will help you learn this new skill. The best way to use the script is to read it into a tape recorder, or have a friend whose voice you enjoy do it for you. Then you can simply listen to the tape on a regular basis. The script is to be read in a calm, pleasant voice, and the pace should be unhurried. The reader should pause frequently. The pauses are indicated by a series of dots (. . .). In fact, it is extremely helpful if the words can be adapted to the natural rhythm of your breathing, so that the talking occurs as you exhale, and the silences take place as you inhale. It is recommended that you practice once a day for the first few weeks, until relaxation becomes a more automatic response.

Always begin by finding a comfortable place to sit or lie down—

a quiet place where you will not be disturbed. Loosen any clothing that may be binding you, and make sure that your arms, hands, and legs are uncrossed.

Relaxation Script

When you are seated comfortably, close your eyes and begin by taking a deep breath, inhaling energy and clarity . . . and then exhaling tension. . . . Once again, a deep breath, inhaling energy . . . and exhaling tension. . . . Now, allow yourself to establish a comfortable, rhythmic pattern of breathing. . . . As you begin to focus on your breathing, imagine that there is a balloon right behind your belly button. As you inhale, the balloon fills with air . . . and as you exhale the balloon flattens out. . . . Let your stomach become relaxed as you gently inhale . . . and exhale . . . inhale . . . and exhale. . . . Give yourself a moment to enjoy this slow, deep, rhythmic breathing. . . .

Now, allow your attention to focus on your hands. . . . As you continue to breathe slowly and deeply, you will begin to notice a sensation in your hands. . . . It might be a tingling in your palms or fingers, or a feeling of increased warmth, a feeling of heaviness, a slight pulsing, or perhaps some other sensation. . . . That sensation is your body's way of letting you know that it is prepared to move into a more relaxed state. . . . As you remain focused on your hands, you can begin to use your breathing to support this process of relaxation. . . . As you exhale, breathe out any tension you are holding in your hands. . . . Exhale and relax . . . exhale and release. . . . Use each "out breath" to relax your hands just a little bit more. . . . As your hands become more and more relaxed, allow the feeling of relaxation to move past your wrists into the lower parts of your arms, once again exhaling any tension you find there . . . exhale and release . . . continuing to breath slowly and deeply. . . . Let the relaxation move past your elbows into the upper parts of your arms. . . . As you exhale, allow all the tension to flow gently out of those muscles . . . arms relaxed now, feeling long and loose and comfortably heavy. . . .

As you continue breathing slowly and deeply, you can now allow the feeling of relaxation to move over the tops of your shoulders and across to the base of your neck. . . . Breathing out all the tension you have been holding in that area . . . exhale and relax . . . exhale, and allow those muscles to release. . . . You may feel your shoulders drop ever so slightly as those muscles become more and more relaxed. . . . Focusing now on the base of your neck, let the relaxation begin to travel up over the top of your head . . . and as you exhale . . . allow all the muscles in your scalp to relax and release. . . . Imagine your scalp becoming very smooth . . . as smooth as the surface of a mountain lake on a warm summer's day, when the air is very, very still. . . . Continuing to breathe slowly and deeply . . . let the feeling of relaxation move down into your forehead . . . melting away any lines of worry or tension. . . . Now allow the tiny muscles at the corners of your eyes to relax . . . and let your face become very soft and relaxed . . . your cheeks . . . the muscles of your jaw. . . . You may find that your jaw drops slightly as those muscles relax. . . . As you continue to exhale tension, let the feeling of relaxation move down to the muscles in the front of your neck and your throat . . . continuing now into your chest and abdomen . . . breathing slowly and deeply . . . and with every "out-breath" allowing those muscles to become more deeply relaxed. . . .

Focusing once more on the back of your neck, allow the feeling of relaxation to begin moving down your spine, one vertebra at a time. . . . As you move slowly down your spine, exhaling all tension, let the muscles on either side of your spine become comfortably relaxed . . . moving slowly past your shoulders . . . down toward your waist . . . all the way down to the base of your spine. . . . Now, as you continue to breathe slowly and deeply, let this same feeling of relaxation gently flow into your hips and buttocks . . . your genitals . . . and then through your entire pelvis . . . exhaling any tension you find in these muscles . . . and, with every exhalation, becoming even more deeply relaxed. . . .

Now let the feeling of relaxation move down into your thighs, once again exhaling tension . . . supporting the process with your breathing. . . . Allow the relaxation to move past your knees into the lower parts of your legs . . . your shins, your calves . . . so that, as you continue to breathe slowly and deeply, your legs begin to feel comfortably heavy and very relaxed. . . . Let the relaxed feeling move past your ankles now, and into your feet . . . and your toes. . . .

Now take a moment to fully enjoy this comfortable feeling of relaxation . . . allowing each breath to continue to relax you even more fully . . . and appreciating your body for its willingness to respond in this way. . . . Remind yourself that, with practice, you will be able to return to this very relaxed state whenever you wish. . . . (long pause)

Now, knowing that this state of relaxation will be available to you again, you may begin to move back into the present. . . . As I count from one to three, allow yourself gently and gradually to become more alert and aware. . . . One . . . becoming aware of the room, the sounds, the feeling of your body as it is supported in your chair . . . two . . . feeling more awake and alert, your body feeling relaxed and refreshed . . . three . . . feeling wide awake and refreshed, and, when you're ready, open your eyes.

IMAGERY AND THE
INNER CHILD

Once you have learned to respond easily to the relaxation script, you are ready for an imagery experience. What follows is a script that will enable you to visualize your "inner child" and hold a dialogue with her. The first part of the script is designed to lead you back into a state of deep relaxation. You will find that it is much shorter than the script for the deep-relaxation exercise. The assumption is that, if you have been practicing the relaxation technique, you are now able to move into a relaxed state more quickly and easily. If you find that you are having any difficulty with this, you may substitute the slower, more detailed, directions you have been following in the previous script.

Before you begin your adventure in imagery, I would like to stress one important point. An image is not necessarily visual. Some people "hear" their images, and some people "feel" or "sense" them. Unless you know for sure which type of imaging is natural for you, it is best to avoid any expectations. Whatever comes up for you is exactly right.

As before, find a comfortable place to sit or lie down—a place where you will not be disturbed. Make sure that your clothes are not binding you in any noticeable way, and that your hands, arms, and legs are uncrossed.

Inner Child Script

When you are seated comfortably, invite yourself to take a deep, relaxing breath . . . inhaling energy and clarity . . . and exhaling tension. . . . Once again, a deep breath, inhaling energy . . . and exhaling tension. . . . As you focus on your breathing, allow yourself to use each "out breath" to release whatever tension you might be holding anywhere in your body. . . . Imagine that there is a balloon behind your belly button that fills with air when you inhale . . . and gently flattens out as you exhale. . . . Allow your stomach to relax as the balloon first expands . . . and then gently flattens out. . . . Let yourself remain focused on your breathing as your body naturally establishes its own comfortable rhythm . . . inhaling . . . and exhaling . . . inhaling . . . and exhaling. . . .

Now allow yourself to focus on your hands, and let yourself become aware of a slight sensation of tingling, or warmth, or heaviness, or perhaps some other sensation. . . . Recall this sensation as the signal that your body is prepared to move into a state of deep relaxation. . . . And now use your breathing to help your hands become comfortably relaxed . . . using your "out breath" to release any muscle tension you find in your hands. . . . As your hands relax, allow the relaxation to flow past your wrists into your lower arms . . . past your elbows into your upper arms . . . supporting this gentle process of relaxation with your breathing. . . . Now let your shoulders relax, feeling them drop slightly as you exhale any tension you may find in those muscles. . . . Allow this comfortable feeling of relaxation to continue to flow on toward the base of your neck . . . and over the top of your head . . . letting the muscles in your scalp relax . . . moving down into your forehead . . . releasing any lines of tension and worry . . . and paying special attention to the small muscles in the corners of your eyes . . . exhaling tension and allowing those muscles to gently relax. . . . Allow your face to become very soft and relaxed . . . your cheeks . . . jaw muscles . . . and tongue . . . neck . . . and throat. . . .

Focusing now on the back of your neck, and beginning to move down your spine, one vertebra at a time . . . and with every "out breath" releasing tension on either side of your spine, as you move from your neck past your shoulders . . . down past your waist . . . and down to the base of your spine. . . . Relaxation flowing now into your hips and buttocks . . . pelvis and genitals . . . breathing slowly and deeply as you continue to relax and release. . . . Allowing this comfortable feeling of relaxation to move into your thighs . . . exhaling all tension in these muscles . . . and now, past your knees into the lower parts of your legs . . . shins and calves . . . noticing your legs beginning to feel comfortably heavy and more relaxed . . . relaxation moving now past your ankles . . . and into your feet . . . and toes. . . .

Take a moment now, as you continue to breathe slowly and deeply, to enjoy this comfortable state of relaxation . . . allowing every breath to move you gently into an even deeper, more relaxed state. . . .

And now allow an image to form of a perfectly beautiful, peaceful, safe place. . . . It might be a place that you have visited . . . or one that you have read about . . . or dreamed about . . . or a place that you create for yourself right now. . . . And when you have a picture or a sense of this beautiful, safe, and peaceful place, imagine yourself there. . . . Take some time to become aware of the details . . . the sights and colors . . . the sounds and smells . . . the textures. . . . As you look around, find a comfortable place for yourself. . . . Allow yourself to settle down, continuing to observe . . . noticing how calm and serene you feel, as you absorb the peacefulness of this beautiful setting. . . . Take a moment to enjoy this feeling. . . .

When you are ready, allow an image to form of your "inner child" and invite her to join you in this safe place. . . . Let yourself become aware of her appearance, or your sense of her. . . . How old is she? . . . What is she wearing? . . . What does she seem to be feeling? . . . Let her know that you care about her and would like to know more about her needs. . . . Ask her if she would be willing to stay and communicate with you. . . . She may answer you in words, or facial expressions, or feelings, or in some other way. . . . Simply allow yourself to be open and receptive to her. . . . Ask her if there is something you can give her at this time . . . something she needs or would like to have from you. . . . Take some time to interact with her in a loving way. . . . (long pause)

Now ask your "inner child" if there is something you can do differently in your life that will make her feel safer or more secure. . . . If she has an answer for you, imagine yourself putting that information to use. . . . Share these images or ideas with your "inner child," and notice any reactions she might have. . . .

Ask her if she has anything more to share with you at this time. . . . Is there something more you would like her to know? . . . Take a moment to finish these communications. . . . When you both feel complete, let her know that you will be available to be with her again in this safe place. . . . Ask her if there is some way she can let you know when she needs your attention. . . . Find out if there is a particular day or time that she would like to meet with you again. . . . And now, find a place for her—a place where she will feel perfectly safe and comfortable until you get together again. . . . When she is feeling secure, simply allow the image to gently fade away. . . .

Knowing that you can reconnect with this precious "inner child" whenever you wish, you can allow yourself to slowly move back into the present . . . gently becoming more aware . . . bringing with you feelings of relaxation, peace, and well-being. Counting from one to three as you become more aware and alert. . . . One . . . aware of the sounds in the room . . . the feeling of your body as it is supported in your chair. . . . Two. . . . coming back, feeling relaxed and refreshed. . . . And three . . . fully alert and wide awake . . . and when you're ready, open your eyes.

IMAGERY AND THE EXPLORATION OF EMOTIONS

As women move through a breast cancer experience, they sometimes feel overwhelmed by powerful emotions. Depression, anger, and fear are cited most often, although resentment, envy, grief, and sadness are also quite common. These feelings are normal and only become a problem when they cause a woman to feel immobilized or out of control. Usually, this type of reaction is a direct result of not understanding feelings well and trying in every possible way to escape from them or make them go away. Women may resist their feelings in the belief that focusing on them will only make them stronger. They hold back tears because they fear that if they start to cry they will never be able to stop. Actually, this is not the case. A feeling will persist until it is attended to. The truth is that, when it comes to feelings, evasion doesn't work! We tend to be most successful with our emotional selves when we are willing to explore our feelings fully, making a concerted effort to understand the communications we are receiving from within.

The script that follows offers you a way to use imagery as a means to explore and hold a dialogue with an emotion that is causing you concern. Once again, I would like to remind you to free yourself of any expectations. Images are not necessarily visual. Some people "hear" their images, and other people "feel" or "sense" them. Also, images that arise are often unexpected. As the images form, simply allow them to be there without judging them or trying to change them.

As I have mentioned before, the more relaxed you are, the greater your access to the creative part of your mind—the part that is the source of the images that will be unfolding. The beginning of this script will provide you with an opportunity to move into a state of relaxation. Although this segment is somewhat shorter than the deep-relaxation script in the Supplement, it should prove quite comfortable for those people who have already become familiar with relaxation techniques. However, if you find that you require more time or more detailed guidance, please feel free to substitute as much as you wish from the deep-relaxation script.

Find a comfortable place to sit or lie down where you will not be disturbed. Make sure that your clothes are not binding you in any way, and that your hands, arms, and legs are uncrossed.

Exploring Emotions Script

When you are seated comfortably, allow your eyes to close and let yourself take a deep, relaxing breath . . . inhaling energy and clarity . . . and exhaling tension. . . . Once again, take a deep breath, inhaling energy . . . and exhaling tension . . . noticing that every "out breath" becomes an invitation for your body to let go of tension . . . relax and release. . . . As you allow yourself to focus on your breathing, imagine that there is a balloon just behind your belly button. . . . As you inhale, it fills with air . . . and as you exhale, the balloon gently flattens out. . . . Hold the image of that balloon in your mind for a moment . . . filling . . . and flattening . . . as you continue to inhale . . . and exhale . . . letting your stomach relax . . . breathing slowly and deeply . . . and allowing your breathing to find its own comfortable rhythm. . . .

Now let your attention focus on your hands . . . and you will begin to notice a sensation there . . . a slight tingling or a feeling of increased warmth . . . a sense of heaviness, or perhaps some other feeling. . . . This sensation is a signal from your body that it is prepared to move into a state of deep relaxation. . . . Using your breathing to support the process of relaxation, exhale any tension you might be holding in your hands. . . . As your hands become more comfortable, allow the feeling of relaxation to flow past your wrists and into the lower parts of your arms . . . past your elbows and into your upper arms . . . exhaling and releasing . . . noticing that your arms begin to feel long and heavy and very comfortably relaxed. . . .

Allow the feeling of relaxation to move over your shoulders and around to the back of your neck . . . continuing to breathe slowly and deeply as those muscles relax . . . exhaling and releasing. . . . Now let the relaxation move up over the top of your head . . . your scalp becoming very relaxed . . . and down to your forehead . . . using each "out breath" to gently release any lines of worry or tension. . . . Let your face become very soft and relaxed . . . the tiny muscles in the corners of your eyes . . . your cheeks . . . jaw . . . tongue . . . neck and throat. . . . Let the feeling of relaxation flow down to your chest and abdomen . . . breathing out any tension you find there, and letting your body become even more relaxed. . . .

Starting now at the back of your neck, allow the relaxation to move slowly down your back . . . one vertebra at a time . . . muscles on either side of your spine gently releasing and relaxing . . . from your neck . . . down past your shoulders . . . continuing down past your waist . . . all the way down to the base of your spine. . . . Breathing slowly and deeply, let the feeling of relaxation flow into your hips and buttocks . . . your pelvis and genitals . . . inviting those muscles to let go of any tension. . . . Focusing now on your thighs . . . exhaling and releasing as those muscles relax. . . . Moving down past your knees and into the lower part of your legs . . . your shins . . . calves. . . . Continuing to support the process of relaxation with your breathing . . . allowing the relaxation to move past your ankles, into your feet . . . and your toes. . . .

Take a moment now to enjoy this relaxed and comfortable feeling, as your body becomes even more relaxed with each breath. . . .

As you continue to become more and more comfortable, allow an image to form of a safe and lovely place . . . a place you may have been before, or a place that is new . . . one you may have seen or read about, or a place that you create for yourself now . . . and take some time to find a special place for yourself in this secure and beautiful setting. . . . Begin to observe some of the details . . . colors . . . sounds . . . textures. . . . As you breathe, notice how the peace and serenity of this place seem to fill you. . . .

When you're ready, allow an image to form that represents the feeling or emotion you would like to explore. . . . Simply wait for an image to appear and let it be with you in your safe place. . . . Your image may be a person or an animal . . . something in nature like a rock, a tree, or even the wind . . . a character from a fairy tale . . . or perhaps some kind of energy. . . . No matter what form your image takes, allow it to be there with you. . . . Observe it carefully. . . . What are its important features? . . . What is it doing? . . . How do you feel as you study the image? . . . Are you standing a comfortable distance from it? . . . Do you need to move farther away for now? . . . Do you need to get closer? . . .

Tell the image that you are interested in learning more about it, and ask if it would be willing to communicate with you. . . . It may answer you in words or gestures, or you may just get a sense of what it has to say. . . . Let yourself be receptive and open to whatever comes. . . . Explain your feelings to the image and let it know about the difficulties you have been experiencing. . . . Ask if it can give you some insight into why it has been such a disturbing presence in your life. . . . Find out if it needs to make you aware of something that may have escaped you until now. . . . Take some time now to have a dialogue with the image. . . . (long pause)

Ask the image if there is something you can do to experience relief from the emotion that has been of concern to you. . . . If so, imagine how you might use that information in your everyday life. . . . Ask the image if it would be willing to meet with you again so that you can continue to explore together. . . . Notice any changes in the image that may have occurred during your dialogue. . . .

At this point, thank the image for meeting with you in your safe place, and for any insights it may have offered you. . . . Ask if it has anything else it needs you to know at this time. . . . When your communication is complete, allow the image to gently fade. . . .

Knowing that you can continue to explore and to have a dialogue with your image whenever you wish, you can allow yourself to begin, slowly and gently, to move back into the present . . . remembering all that you have learned and experienced in your encounter with it. . . . Counting now from one to three as you become more aware and alert . . . one . . . becoming aware of the sounds in the room . . . the feeling of your body as it is supported in your chair . . . two . . . coming back feeling relaxed and refreshed . . . and three . . . fully alert and wide awake . . . and when you're ready, open your eyes. . . .

APPENDICES

a p p e n d i x   a

□

SUGGESTED READINGS

Andrews, Lynn V. *Medicine Woman*. New York: Harper & Row, 1981.

John-Roger, and McWilliams, Peter. *You Can't Afford the Luxury of a Negative Thought: A Book for People with Any Life-Threatening Illness—Including Life*. Los Angeles: Prelude Press, 1988.

Kübler-Ross, Elisabeth. *On Death and Dying*. New York: Macmillan Publishing Co., 1969.

Kushner, Harold S. *When Bad Things Happen to Good People*. New York: Schocken Books, 1981.

Millman, Dan. *Way of the Peaceful Warrior*. Tiburon, California: H. J. Kramer, Inc., 1984.

Moody, Raymond A., M.D. *Life After Life*. New York: Bantam Books, 1976.

Peck, M. Scott, M.D. *The Road Less Traveled*. New York: Simon and Schuster, 1978.

Rodegast, Pat, and Stanton, Judith. *Emmanuel's Book: A Manual for Living Comfortably in the Cosmos*. New York: Bantam Books, 1987.

Rossman, Martin L., M.D. *Healing Yourself: A Step-by-Step Program for Better Health Through Imagery*. New York: Pocket Books, 1987.

Siegel, Bernie S., M.D. *Love, Medicine and Miracles.* New York: Harper & Row, 1986.
———. *Peace, Love and Healing.* New York: Harper & Row, 1989.
Spingarn, Natalie Davis. *Hanging in There: Living Well on Borrowed Time.* New York: Stein and Day, 1984.

a p p e n d i x   b

□

PERSONAL CONNECTIONS, SUPPORT, AND COUNSELING

Reach to Recovery

This is a program run by your local branch of the American Cancer Society. Reach to Recovery volunteers are women who have had breast cancer and have been trained to offer support and information to newly diagnosed breast cancer patients. Both hospital and home visits are part of the services offered. Hospital visits must be arranged by a physician. Home visits can be requested by the patient. Consult your telephone directory for a local unit, or call the Chartered Division in your state for the location of the unit nearest you. For further information, contact the national office:

> American Cancer Society
> Tower Place
> 3340 Peachtree Road, NE
> Atlanta, GA 30026
> (404) 320-3333

Your local unit will also have information available on breast cancer support groups in the area as well as names and locations of shops where you can purchase a breast prosthesis.

Y-ME

This is a national nonprofit breast cancer information and support organization headquartered in the Chicago area. Services include both a toll-free and a twenty-four-hour hot line providing cancer information and referrals and emotional support. Trained staff and volunteers, most of whom have had breast cancer, are available to answer questions. Upon request, volunteers are matched as closely as possible with the caller with regard to age, marital status, and type of treatment. Y-ME also sponsors monthly support meetings in the Chicago area and in other states where Y-ME chapters operate. Call or write to:

> Y-ME National Organization for Breast Cancer
>   Information and Support
> 18220 Harwood Avenue
> Homewood, IL 60430
> (800) 221-2141 (9 A.M. to 5 P.M. CST)
> (708) 799-8228 (24 hours)

The YWCA Encore Program

This program was designed to provide supportive discussion and rehabilitative exercise for women who have been treated for breast cancer. To find the location of the program nearest you, contact:

> YWCA Encore Program
> YWCA National Headquarters
> 726 Broadway
> New York, NY 10003
> (212) 614-2827

The National Coalition for Cancer Survivorship

NCCS is a national network of independent groups and individuals concerned with survivorship issues and sources of support for cancer patients and their families. The organization facilitates communication between people involved with cancer survivorship, promotes peer support, serves as an information clearinghouse, and advocates the interest of cancer survivors. For information, contact:

NCCS
323 Eighth Street SW
Albuquerque, NM 87102
(505) 764-9956

Hospitals

Many of the larger hospitals run support groups for breast cancer patients. Contact a staff social worker or the Department of Patient Services.

Phone Book

Look in the White Pages under "Cancer" for a listing of organizations, some of which may provide emotional support for cancer patients.

INFORMATION RESOURCES

National Cancer Institute

The Cancer Information Service (CIS) is a nationwide toll-free telephone program sponsored by the National Cancer Institute. Trained information specialists are available to answer questions about cancer from the public, cancer patients and their families, and health professionals. To be automatically connected to the CIS office serving your area, call:

1-800-4-CANCER

In Alaska, call 1-800-638-6070; in Hawaii, on Oahu, call 524-1234 (on neighboring islands, call collect).

You can obtain free copies of an excellent series of pamphlets published by NCI, entitled the Breast Cancer Patient Education Series by calling CIS or writing to:

Office of Cancer Communications
National Cancer Institute
Building 31, Room 10A24
Bethesda, MD 20892

In addition, NCI has published a paperback handbook called *The Breast Cancer Digest: A Guide to Medical Care, Emotional Support,*

Educational Programs and Resources. It is an excellent book which provides background information on all aspects of breast cancer, including detection, diagnosis, treatment, rehabilitation, psychosocial impact, and resources for patients and families. Although it has not been updated since 1984, it is still generally accurate, and contains comprehensive information. *The Breast Cancer Digest* is available free of charge, and may be ordered as follows:

> U.S. Department of Health and Human Services
> Public Health Service
> National Institutes of Health
> NCI
> Bethesda, MD 20205
> request NIH publication number: 84-1691

National Alliance of Breast Cancer Organizations

NABCO is a not-for-profit central resource that provides individuals and health organizations with accurate, up-to-date information on all aspects of breast cancer and promotes affordable detection and treatment. The organization is also active in efforts to influence public and private health policy on issues that directly pertain to breast cancer, such as insurance reimbursement and health care legislation. NABCO has published the extensive *Breast Cancer Resource List*, describing a multitude of books, pamphlets, organizations and other resources of value to the breast cancer patient and her family. To order the resource list or to obtain current information pertaining to breast cancer diagnosis and/or treatment, contact:

> NABCO
> 2nd Floor
> 1180 Avenue of the Americas
> New York, NY 10036
> (212) 719-0154

AN OVERVIEW OF BREAST CANCER DIAGNOSIS AND TREATMENT

The cell is the basic building block of the body. Cells reproduce and grow in an orderly fashion, and as they mature, they take on the characteristics and functions of our various tissues or organs. An organ is a collection of specialized cells organized to perform one or more important body functions (e.g., liver, lung, heart, breast). In an organ, cancer starts with abnormal cells that do not mature properly. They begin to reproduce in an uncontrolled way, overgrowing the normal cells. If left untreated, these cells can spread to other parts of the body where they will establish colonies of cancer cells called **metastases**. To date, we do not know why cancer cells begin to grow in the breast. There are many theories implicating diet, heredity, environment, and stress, but the truth is that no theory has yet been proved. The cause may very well be a combination of many factors, some of which are as yet unknown.

While we do not know how to prevent breast cancer, we do know how to detect it. We also know that the earlier it is found, the more curable it is. There are two ways that breast cancer can be detected. One is with a breast X ray, called a **mammogram**. Using this technique, a cancer can be found when it is extremely tiny, long before it can actually be felt as a lump in the breast. The other method is through examination, either by the woman herself (**breast self-examination**) or by her physician (**clinical examination**).

If the doctor sees anything suspicious, either on the X ray or on physical examination of the breast, he/she will order a **biopsy**. A biopsy is the removal of a sample of the breast tissue thought to be abnormal so it can be examined under the microscope. This biopsy is usually done by a surgeon or a surgical **oncologist** (cancer specialist). There are two major ways that the tissue may be removed. One is a **needle biopsy**. In this procedure, a needle is inserted into the lump, and fluid is withdrawn. The fluid is then examined under the microscope for the presence of cancer cells. The second common approach is an **excisional biopsy**. With this technique, surgery is performed, and the lump itself is removed. With either method, the tissue sampled will be carefully reviewed by a **pathologist** (a physician who specializes in the study of disease by examination of tissue and body fluids). The pathology report will usually determine whether or not a woman needs treatment for breast cancer. Frequently, a biopsy turns out to be **negative**, meaning that it was a false alarm and the tissue was **benign** (noncancerous). For the purposes of this book, however, we will consider the steps that are taken when the report is **positive**—that is, when the diagnosis is cancer.

Sometimes, cancer is detected so early that no further treatment is needed other than removal of the **malignant** (cancerous) tissue during biopsy. In most cases, further treatment is necessary. The next step is usually surgery, of which there are basically two types: **lumpectomy** (removal of the lump) or **mastectomy** (removal of the entire breast). Mastectomy used to be the only option available to the breast cancer patient. In certain situations, it may still be the treatment of choice, or the only choice available. It is important for a woman facing this surgery to know that breast reconstruction is now an alternative to be considered either at the time of surgery or at some future date. Reconstruction is performed by a plastic surgeon. The other procedure, **lumpectomy** or **partial mastectomy**, is relatively new. It can be performed subject to certain conditions having to do with the size and location of the lump, the particular type of breast cancer, and whether or not there are multiple tumors

in the breast. The surgeon will remove the lump and some surrounding tissue (**margins**), if this has not already been performed
at the time of the biopsy. The remainder of the breast will be left
intact. This procedure is almost always followed by radiation therapy.

With either surgical approach, the lymph nodes under the arm
will usually be removed (**axillary lymph node dissection**). The
lymph nodes are simply what most of us know as glands—like the
ones in the neck that may be swollen when we are sick. The lym-
phatic system is part of the body's circulatory system. When breast
cancer cells begin to spread (**metastasize**) out of the breast, they are
often discovered first in the lymph nodes under the arm. After these
nodes are removed, they will be examined by the pathologist. Discovering whether there are cancer cells present in the lymph nodes
gives the physician some very important information about what
kind of follow-up treatment might be needed after surgery.

Before treatment is undertaken, the newly diagnosed breast cancer
patient may be asked to undergo several tests. The most common
ones are a chest X ray, bone scan, liver scan, and brain scan. While
these tests may sound frightening, they are not painful, although
some of them might be quite time-consuming. They enable the
doctor to determine whether cancer has spread to any of those areas.
In addition, there will be a panel of blood tests which provide other
information. One test, which must be performed by the pathologist
at the time he/she examines the malignant tissue from the biopsy,
is called a **hormone receptor test**. Estrogen and progesterone, two
hormones that are naturally produced by women, are necessary for
the growth of normal breast tissue. The hormones are attracted to
breast cells due to the action of **hormone receptors**. These receptors
are really chemicals that sit on the surface of the cells. The chemicals
not only bind the hormones, but also help them pass through the
cell wall into the interior of the cell. Some breast cancers, called
hormone receptor positive, keep this property of normal breast
tissue. They, too, have receptors that bind hormones and help them
pass into the cell's interior. Breast cancers that are receptor positive
become more active in the presence of estrogen/progesterone, and

tend to die off in their absence. The presence or absence of hormone receptors in the breast cancer tissue will influence what type of further treatment may be recommended after lumpectomy or mastectomy.

After all the tests and reports have been completed, each individual case needs to be reviewed by a competent physician, usually a **medical oncologist** (an internist who has specialized in cancer). At that time some recommendation will be made as to whether any further treatment is necessary. If so, it would be radiation therapy, chemotherapy, hormone therapy, or some combination of these. **Radiation therapy**, which uses high-energy beams like X rays or gamma rays, destroys cancer cells in a specific area (**local treatment**). One of its important uses is to mop up any stray cancer cells that might remain in the breast after a lumpectomy. This treatment is supervised by a **radiation oncologist**, a physician who specializes in the use of radiation for the treatment of cancer. **Chemotherapy** is treatment with cancer-killing chemicals that are taken into the body orally, intramuscularly, or intravenously, in case there is a chance that cancer has spread to an area outside the breast. The chemicals are absorbed by the rapidly growing cancer cells and interfere with their growth and reproduction. **Hormone therapy** is the use of medication to prevent the stimulation of breast cancer cells by estrogen and/or progesterone in those cases where the cancer is known to be hormone receptor positive. Supervised by the medical oncologist, hormonal treatments and chemotherapy drugs circulate in the bloodstream and are given to kill cancer cells anywhere in the body (**systemic treatment**). Such treatment therefore adds to the effects of radiation and surgery, which treat only a specific area. It is important that every individual case be evaluated for both local and systemic treatment, thus assuring each breast cancer patient of her best chance for cure.

appendix e

□

QUESTIONS TO ASK THE DOCTOR AT THE TIME OF DIAGNOSIS

Diagnosis

1. How do you know for sure that I have breast cancer?
2. Will I need any (further) tests to determine my treatment options?

      If so, what are they and when can they be done?

Treatment Options

1. Will I need (further) surgery?
   If not, why not?
2. Do I have a choice of what kind of surgery I will have?
   If not, why not?
   If so, please explain my options.
3. Do you have an opinion as to which choice is better?
   If so, please explain.
   If not, how do I make such a difficult choice?

4. How much time do I have to make a decision?

5. How can I arrange to get a second opinion?

Lumpectomy

1. Will you describe the procedure?

2. What are the advantages, disadvantages, risks, and complications?

3. How will I look after surgery?

4. How long does recovery take, and what can I expect in terms of pain or discomfort?

5. When would I be able to go back to work?

6. Will I need radiation therapy?

   If not, why not?

   If so (please see section on Radiation Therapy)

7. Will my lymph nodes be removed?

   If not, why not?

   If so (please see section on Lymph Node Dissection)

Radiation Therapy

1. What does this kind of therapy do?

2. Is it safe?

3. Are there any risks or side effects?

4. When and where will treatment take place?

5. How long will radiation therapy take?

6. Will I be radioactive?

7. Will I be able to work while I am receiving treatment?

8. If I should need a mastectomy at some time in the future, will radiation affect my chances to have breast reconstruction?

   If so, in what way?

Mastectomy (modified radical)

1. Will you describe the procedure?
2. What are the advantages, disadvantages, risks, and complications?
3. How will I look after surgery? Can you show me any pictures?
4. Where can I get information on purchasing a breast prosthesis, and how soon after surgery can I buy one? What will I do in the meantime?
5. How long does recovery take, and what can I expect in terms of pain or discomfort?
6. When will I be able to return to work?
7. Am I a candidate for immediate breast reconstruction?
    If not, why not? What are other options for reconstruction?
    If so, can we arrange for a plastic surgeon to be present at the time of the mastectomy?
8. Will you refer me to a plastic surgeon for a consultation before my mastectomy?
9. Will I need radiation therapy?
    If not, why not?
    If so (please see section on Radiation Therapy)
10. Will my lymph nodes be removed?
    If not, why not?
    If so (please see section on Lymph Node Dissection)

Lymph Node Dissection

1. What are lymph nodes, and why are they important in breast cancer diagnosis and treatment?
2. Will my lymph nodes be removed?
    If not, why not?
3. When will this surgery be performed?
4. Are there any risks, side effects, or complications?

5. How long does recovery take, and what can I expect in terms of pain or discomfort?

6. How will the surgery affect my arm movement, and who will give me a set of exercises?

7. In what way will microscopic examination of my lymph nodes help to determine further treatment?

Postsurgical Treatment

1. Will I need any further treatment after surgery?

   If not, why not?

   If so, what might the treatment(s) be?

2. Would a consultation with a medical oncologist be advisable at that time?

   If not, why not?

   If so, can you recommend one?

Chemotherapy

1. How do we decide whether or not I will need chemotherapy?
2. What does chemotherapy do?
3. How and where is it administered?
4. How often would I be receiving treatment?
5. What are the possible side effects and complications?
6. Will chemotherapy make me sick?

   If so, are there medications that will alleviate some of the side effects?

7. Will I lose my hair?
8. Will I be able to work while I am receiving chemotherapy?
9. How long will the course of treatment be?

Hormone Therapy

1. What is hormone therapy, and why is it effective in controlling or curing breast cancer?
2. What are hormone receptor tests?
3. Have my hormone receptor tests been done yet?
    If not, why not? When will they be done?
    If so, are the results positive or negative, and what do the results mean?
4. Will I need hormone therapy?
5. How is hormone therapy administered?
6. How long will I have to continue with it?
7. Are there any side effects or risks?

Emotional Support

1. Would you contact the American Cancer Society to arrange for a hospital visit from a Reach to Recovery volunteer?
2. Do you know of any breast cancer support groups in the area?
    If not, where can I find that information?
3. Can you put me in touch with any of your patients who have had this type of treatment and are already recovered?

appendix f

□

A REVIEW OF BREAST RECONSTRUCTION TECHNIQUES

Breast reconstruction is the surgical restoration of the breast contour, nipple, and areola (the dark area surrounding the nipple). There are two basic approaches to breast reconstruction following mastectomy. The first utilizes an artificial implant, which is a type of silicone sac filled with silicone gel and/or saline. In most cases, the implant is inserted into a pocket created behind the chest muscle at the mastectomy site, resulting in a reconstructed breast mound. This is by far the simplest procedure, and is normally available to women who have sufficient skin and muscle in the area where the mastectomy was performed to provide adequate coverage for the implant.

When the skin and muscle remaining after a mastectomy are very tight, a variation of the implant procedure can be used. The first step in this method involves the insertion of a temporary, expandable implant (**tissue expander**). At the time that it is placed behind the muscle in the chest wall, the expander is fairly flat. Over a period of weeks or months, the plastic surgeon gradually inflates it by injecting saline through a valve that is left under the skin, thus allowing the existing tissue to stretch. Once the expander has reached the appropriate size and the tissue has been stretched adequately, it is replaced with a permanent implant.

The other type of procedure involves transferring a flap of the woman's skin, muscle, and fat tissue, along with its own blood supply, to the chest where it is then shaped into a breast. The flap is taken from a donor site somewhere on the body. The donor sites include upper back or side (**latissimus dorsi flap**), the lower abdomen (**trans rectus abdominus muscle flap**, also called a **TRAM flap**), and buttock (**gluteal flap**). The latissimus dorsi flap is used in conjunction with an artificial implant when additional tissue is needed for coverage and a better cosmetic result. The TRAM flap and the gluteal flap usually provide enough tissue so that a woman's breast(s) can be reconstructed without the use of an artificial implant.

Regardless of the method of surgery elected, it can be followed by reconstruction of the nipple and areola. Ordinarily, a plastic surgeon will prefer to wait a few months after the initial reconstruction is completed before restoring the nipple-areola complex. This allows the reconstructed breast to settle and assume its permanent position, and helps to insure a more accurate positioning of the nipple and areola. In some cases, the plastic surgeon can reconstruct the nipple and areola by borrowing tissue from the remaining breast. If that is not possible, the areola is generally reconstructed by taking a skin graft from the upper inner thigh, the back of the ear, or, less commonly, the labial area of the vagina. These tissues are used because, when transplanted, their color darkens and tends to create a more natural effect. A graft is also used to recreate a nipple, with tissue taken from the remaining nipple, the ear lobe, the upper thigh, or the labial area. Sometimes, the surgeon will use tissue from the reconstructed breast itself to form a new nipple. There is also a new technique being used for nipple/areola reconstruction. It involves scarring and tattooing the breast skin. This simple and painless procedure does not necessitate the borrowing of tissue from a donor site and the results are quite remarkable. It may be surprising to discover that not all women are interested in this final phase of the reconstructive process. Some feel that restoration of the breast contour alone is sufficient, and find no compelling reason to continue with further surgery.

If a woman has had bilateral mastectomies (removal of both breasts), her two reconstructed breasts are likely to match. However, when one of her natural breasts remains, matching and symmetry become important issues. When a breast is very large, reconstructing a matching breast can be extremely difficult. In this case, a flap must be used instead of, or in addition to, an implant. Even if the remaining breast is of small to moderate size, the reconstructed breast may not match in fullness, projection, or degree of relaxation. If a woman finds the idea of asymmetry or mismatch very disturbing, she always has the option of having her natural breast surgically revised, either by having it made larger (**augmentation**), smaller (**reduction**), or by having it lifted (**mastopexy**).

Each type of surgery has its advantages and disadvantages. The simple implant procedure requires a relatively uncomplicated type of surgery, and recovery time is fairly rapid. The major postsurgical complication is the excessive formation of scar tissue around the implant (**capsular contracture**), which can make the reconstructed breast feel hard and can sometimes cause considerable pain. Correcting that condition may require additional surgery. The abdominal and gluteal flap procedures utilize the woman's own tissue, often eliminating the need to introduce any foreign substance into the body. Reconstruction that uses either of these flaps is especially desirable when a woman is large-breasted, has insufficient tissue left at the mastectomy site, or has undergone radiation therapy to the chest area. If the TRAM flap is used, the patient winds up with a tummy tuck in addition to her reconstructed breast(s), and many women feel that this is a very worthwhile bonus. However, the flap procedures are far more complex than a simple implant insertion, and involve heavier, lengthier surgery. As a result, the patient will spend a considerably longer time under anesthesia. Because the surgery is more extensive, the recovery period tends to be significantly longer, and the possibilities for complications are greater.

Breast reconstruction may be performed at the time of a mastectomy, or anywhere from a few days to many years later. Today, every woman who must undergo a mastectomy deserves to be told about breast reconstruction prior to her surgery, allowing her time to collect information and make some decisions. Many doctors feel that a better cosmetic result is obtained when the tissue at the mastectomy site is first allowed to heal and soften. They will, therefore, often advise a three- to six-month delay before breast reconstruction is performed. However, surgical techniques are constantly being refined, and immediate reconstruction has become much more popular in recent years. Generally speaking, the simple implant procedure, with or without a tissue expander, is the one that is most often considered for immediate reconstruction. Most, although not all, plastic surgeons believe that the flap procedures are not ideal for immediate reconstruction because they subject the breast cancer patient to too much surgery and anesthesia all at one time.

Breast reconstruction should only be performed by a board-certified plastic surgeon. He/she will evaluate each case on an individual basis to determine the most suitable type of procedure as well as the most favorable timing for surgery.*

* For a comprehensive presentation of all aspects of breast reconstruction written for the layperson, I highly recommend *A Woman's Decision: Breast Care, Treatment, and Reconstruction,* by Karen Berger and John Bostwick III, M.D., St. Louis, Missouri: The C. V. Mosby Company, 1984.